"He has drive and energy; he is likely to have been popular and made a name for himself at college in sports as well as in academic subjects; he might have been a team captain. He marries early, works hard, and takes on responsibility. He is restless and active, and his mood swings between anxiety and boredom, but he cannot spare time for exercise or relaxation. His only recreation is eating and drinking. He drives fast. He has business lunches and work to take home on weekends."

WITH THIS BOOK YOU CAN WIN.

If you don't want to die young you must consider not only the killers that are general, but particularly the pitfalls for someone like you. Outwitting your deadliest enemies is not a dull routine. Armed with knowledge and intelligence, it is a game of skill—and a game you can surely win.

—

HOW NOT TO DIE YOUNG
was originally published by Stein and Day.

How Not to Die Young

DR. JOAN GOMEZ

PUBLISHED BY POCKET BOOKS NEW YORK

HOW NOT TO DIE YOUNG

Stein and Day edition published 1972

POCKET BOOK edition published October, 1973

This POCKET BOOK edition includes every word
contained in the original, higher-priced edition. It is printed
from brand-new plates made from completely reset, clear, easy-to-read
type. POCKET BOOK editions are published by POCKET BOOKS, a division
of Simon & Schuster, Inc., 630 Fifth Avenue, New York, N.Y. 10020.
Trademarks registered in the United States and other countries.

L

Contents

How Not to
Die Young

1

Evidence You May Choose to Ignore

1. LEWIS, Samuel S. Suddenly on June 16. Loving husband of Ruth, father of David, Leo and Sarah. Aged 45 years. Sadly missed. Services "Park West" June 22 at 2 P.M. In lieu of flowers contributions may be sent to the Heart Fund.

2. BUTLER, Walter L. After a long illness, bravely borne. Husband of Roslyn, Father of Eileen and Jonathan. Service and interment in Cleveland, Ohio.

3. STOCK. On Friday, June 18th, 1972, as the result of a motor accident, Philip Raymond Stock, aged 21. Darling son of Elizabeth and brother of James and Stephen. Funeral service Wednesday June 23rd, 3 P.M., Clare College Chapel, Cambridge.

4. REYNOLDS. On June 17th, 1972, after a short illness in hospital, Caroline Mary, wife of Dr. Hugh Reynolds, 51 Belvedere Grove, Wimbledon, S.W. 19, mother of Peter and Paul. Funeral private. No flowers. No letters. All donations to the Imperial Cancer Research Fund.

Any of your friends in the roundup list? It's like a dead eel slithering down the inside of your collar when it's someone you know. Sam, for instance. They said some nice things about him at the next board meeting, which he'd have liked hearing if he'd been around; and there's to be some kind of handout to the widow. But Sam's the one who's missing out. He'll never see his kids grow up, he won't be at his sons' graduation day, nor be on hand when young Sally starts having boyfriends. The Reynolds twins aren't going to relish it much, either, now that their mother has left them more absolutely than by divorce. It'll mean their going away to school at age twelve and spending their vacations between their grandparents and an aunt who feels more duty than love toward them.

As for Wally, he went through hell before he got his. It wasn't fun for his family watching it happen, either.

Young Philip had everything before him, for this had been his last term at Cambridge. He's missed all the useful, pleasurable years of work and achievement, sunshine and sex, living . . .

These four died before they'd had their share, like the 200,000 men and 121,000 women between fifteen and fifty-five who will die in the next year in the United States, and the 37,000 men and 22,000 women of the same age range whose number will be up in Britain. You think it couldn't happen to you? You are made of the same stuff, live in the same Western so-called civilization. But if you would rather not know and recognize the dangers, shut your eyes for the next few pages and take particular care, wherever you are, not to look at any life tables; say that statistics are all lies, that the Metropolitan Life Insurance Company is not in business for profit and takes no care that its figures are accurate; that the demographic reports put out by WHO (World Health Organization) are hooey; and that the Registrar General in Britain doesn't know a birth from a death.

But you may prefer to know your enemies, and from your knowledge defeat them. None of those four people need have died young.

You might think that living in the richest country in the world, the one with the "mostest" in medical research and technical advancement, you are safe enough; or you might imagine that you are, healthwise, in clover too, if you live in Britain, where there has been a comprehensive health service for more than twenty years, providing free medical treatment for all; in and out of hospital; from lights-up to curtains, with rehabilitation and convalescent holidays to top it off. In either of these countries you would expect to be sure of living out the scriptural three score years and ten, at least. You would be wrong.

We have made dramatic advances in our knowledge of the sciences, including physiology, psychology, and medicine itself. In the last hundred years there have been more medical discoveries than in all the preceding centuries put together. Grab a handful of the biggest plums: anesthetics and the techniques of antisepsis and, later, asepsis, making surgery not only possible but popular; microbiology and the work of Pasteur, immortalized on every carton of milk; mass immunization, from smallpox to polio to measles; Freud and his theories, to today's tidal wave of tranquilizers; X rays, beginning with Roentgen's paper in 1895; sulfa drugs, dating from Domagk's painstaking work in 1935 (it has been said that World War II was won by sulfaguanidine, the Jeep, and the DC-3); and penicillin, discovered and developed between 1929 and 1939 by Fleming, Florey, Heatley, and Chain.

Diagnostic instruments like the electrocardiograph, undreamed of a hundred years ago, are common today. Insulin and the tablet method of controlling diabetes have both been discovered in this century. Steroids began their therapeutic revolution in 1949; there is the current craze for "spare-part" surgery; machines to take over for diseased kidneys; ultrasonics in obstetrics, and lasers in ophthalmology. Every year brings a breakthrough of some sort, and almost every year in the United States a new institute is founded, devoted primarily to research. Discoveries in the last few years include cromoglycate for the prevention of asthmatic attacks (Britain), clomiphene to give the infertile female babies galore, L-dopa for Parkinson's disease, hypotensive drugs to take the blood pressure down a notch, and a spate of new antibiotics to keep one step ahead of developing bacterial resistance to the oldies.

Social improvements have done as much for health as purely medical advances. In our part of the world, poverty, starvation, squalor, and the spread of infection through unsanitary conditions are problems we have almost completely solved. The bicycle and, since that, other forms of personal transport have done much to provide our race with the vigor of hybridization, after centuries during which the stock was weakened by intermarriage with those within walking distance.

We've come a long way. If you had been born in the days of the glory of Greece your life expectancy would have been thirty years. An American in 1750 had, on average, a thirty-six-year future; a Briton could expect to live thirty-nine years at the time of Waterloo. (See Fig. 1.)

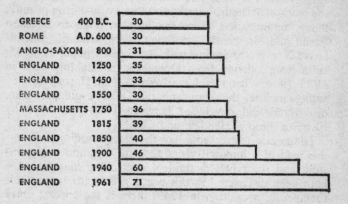

GREECE	400 B.C.	30
ROME	A.D. 600	30
ANGLO-SAXON	800	31
ENGLAND	1250	35
ENGLAND	1450	33
ENGLAND	1550	30
MASSACHUSETTS	1750	36
ENGLAND	1815	39
ENGLAND	1850	40
ENGLAND	1900	46
ENGLAND	1940	60
ENGLAND	1961	71

Figure 1
Diagrammatic Representation of the Average Length of Life from Ancient to Recent Times

Now take a look at what killed people in England and Wales a hundred years ago. (Fig. 2.)

The worst enemies were TB of the lungs (phthisis), scarlet fever, and diarrhea. How many of your friends have been erased by these troubles today? None, I'd guess. The devastating epidemics of infectious fevers are over and done; motherhood is safer than crossing the street;

Figure 2
England and Wales: Annual Death Rates from Various Causes Per Million Living

CAUSES OF DEATH	5 Years 1861-65.	5 Years 1866-70.	5 Years 1871-75.	5 Years 1876-80.	5 Years 1881-85.	5 Years 1886-90.	5 Years 1891-95.
ALL CAUSES	23582.6	22424.6	21962.4	20791.0	19403.0	18894.6	18737.8
Smallpox	218.6	104.8	410.8	78.4	78.0	15.6	20.0
Measles	456.6	428.4	373.2	384.8	413.0	468.4	487.8
Scarlet Fever	982.4	959.8	758.6	679.6	435.8	240.6	182.4
Typhus	}		81.4	34.2	22.8	6.6	3.8
Enteric Fever	} 921.8	849.8	373.8	277.2	216.0	179.2	173.6
Simple and Ill-defined Fever	}		140.2	69.2	34.2	16.6	8.0
Whooping Cough	515.8	545.0	498.6	527.0	458.6	443.6	396.4
Diphtheria	247.6	126.8	120.8	121.8	156.2	169.8	263.0
Other Miasmatic Diseases	46.0	39.6	25.4	18.4	16.4	45.4	425.0
Cholera	42.4	172.4	30.6	20.4	16.2	14.6	21.4
Diarrhea, Dysentery	874.0	1062.8	1000.4	852.4	855.8	667.0	630.4
Malarial Diseases	16.2	10.0	8.4	7.8	11.4	6.4	3.8
Hydrophobia	9.4	0.8	3.0	1.8	1.2	0.6	0.2
Other Zoogenous Diseases	0.6	1.0	1.2	1.8	2.4	1.8	1.8
Venereal Diseases	77.6	90.8	92.6	95.6	93.4	83.6	79.8
Erysipelas	87.4	82.4	105.6	80.8	82.8	54.2	47.8
Puerperal Fever	56.0	55.6	86.0	81.0	92.6	76.4	76.6
Other Septic Diseases	8.3	14.6	20.8	23.8	23.6	14.6	13.2
Thrush	50.0	49.8	49.8	48.0	29.4	22.0	14.0
Other Parasitic Diseases	8.6	7.6	7.9	9.0	7.2	6.8	4.6
Intemperance	41.6	35.4	37.8	42.4	48.2	56.0	68.0
Other Dietetic Diseases	30.4	26.6	21.2	25.0	15.6	11.4	12.0
Rheumatic Fever, Rheumatism of Heart	} 108.2	115.0	127.2	62.0	97.6	88.2	88.0
Rheumatism	}			77.0	34.8	33.0	31.6
Cancer	367.8	403.8	445.0	493.6	547.0	631.6	712.2
Phthisis	2526.6	2447.8	2913.0	2039.8	1830.4	1635.4	1463.6
Other Tubercular and Scrofulous Diseases	784.4	752.4	722.6	775.0	710.2	687.6	659.8
Diabetes Mellitus	29.2	31.8	35.8	40.4	51.4	62.4	60.4
Other Constitutional Diseases	51.2	63.8	50.6	87.0	108.0	131.0	156.0

The figures for certain diseases prior to 1881 cannot be shown, and for other diseases the figures are only approximate.

birth, too, that four-inch journey through the valley of the
shadow of life, is 300 percent safer than it was even fifty
years ago. The expectation of life for a child born now in
the West is 30 percent better than it was at the beginning
of the century. But neither the United Kingdom nor the
United States, despite the dollars and the know-how, is by
any means the healthiest spot to live. There are thirty
countries where the outlook for survival is better than
Uncle Sam's, eight where it is better than Britain's. Study
Fig. 3. You'd be safer living in Iceland than in London,
or in poverty-stricken Spain than in plush New York.

Figure 3
Male Expectation of Life at Birth in Years by Country
Some Female Expectations in Brackets

Sweden	71.6	(75.7)
Netherlands	71	(75.9)
Norway	71	
Israel	70.9	
Iceland	70.8	(76.2)
Denmark	70.2	
Japan	68.4	
New Zealand	68.4	
United Kingdom	68.3	(74.4)
Canada	68.3	
East Germany	68.3	
Switzerland	68.2	
Ireland	68.1	
Ukraine	68	
Ryukyu Islands	68	
Australia	67.9	
Northern Ireland	67.8	
Bulgaria	67.8	
Czechoslovakia	67.8	
France	67.8	
Belgium	67.7	
Fed. German Rep.	67.6	
Malta	67.5	
Greece	67.4	
Spain	67.3	
Italy	67.2	
Puerto Rico	67	
Hungary	67	
Austria	66.8	
Rhodesia	66.7	
U.S.A.	66.6	(73.8)
Scotland	66.6	

The outlook in our countries is wonderfully improved for the fetus, the infant, the child at school, and the eighty-year-old. But how much better is it for you? If you are a young adult between eighteen and thirty-five, the chances of your dying before your next birthday are a good deal less than they used to be, mainly because of the bacteria that are on the run. But the situation isn't that much rosier for you than for the other groups, and soon you'll be in the risk group anyway. If you are in the thirty-five to fifty-five age bracket yours is the dropout generation: dropout by death.

The death rate for men in the middle years of adulthood is the only age- and sex-specific rate that has not declined in the developed countries.

For you, the dangers of today are as great as the mammoths were to Stone Age man and the unmitigated depredations of war, famine, and disease were to those in the centuries that followed. It's dangerous to be a man today. The British or American female has an average six-year edge on the male at this time—more than it has ever been—and an even greater edge in highly sophisticated countries like Sweden and the Netherlands. Take another glance at Fig. 3 (opposite).

Check some more figures:

*Expectation of Life at Different Ages in the U.S.**

	0	5	10	15	25	35	45	55	60 years
Men	66.7	64	59	54	45	36	27	19	16
Women	73.8	71	66	61	51	42	33	24	20
And in the U.K.									
Men	68.3	65	60	55	46	36	27	19	15
Women	74.4	71	66	61	51	42	32	24	19 years

* Demographic Year Book (U.N., 1968).

The women are the winners all along the line. Take note if you are a man; and if you are a woman and have one of these rare specimens in your home, remember that this is a creature in danger of becoming extinct, like the dinosaur. If you are a married man there's less than one chance in a thousand that your wife will die before you are forty, but the chances of her becoming a widow are two and a half times as great. There is three times the likelihood in the forty to fifty age bracket. That's how come all these rich American widows are touring Europe, while widowers are extremely scarce.

One possible reason for the excess of male deaths is cigarette smoking. Seventy-five percent of men smoke as against 50 percent of women, while 19 percent of men but only 5 percent of women burn more than twenty cigarettes a day. The chances of dying between ages thirty-five and fifty-five are three or four times greater for heavy smokers than for nonsmokers. Cigarette-associated killers include coronary disease, lung cancer, bronchitis, emphysema, and peptic ulcer, all of which are commoner in men today. Increased exposure to road and industrial hazards

Figure 4
Life Expectation

AGE (in years)

	0	1	2	3	4	5	10	15	20	25
United States* Male										
1900-02†	....47.88	54.35	55.31	55.21	54.79	54.22	50.39	46.06	42.03	38.38
1909-11†	....49.86	55.94	56.59	56.33	55.79	55.11	51.07	46.66	42.48	38.59
1919-21†	....55.50	59.47	59.50	58.99	58.33	57.60	53.44	49.05	44.99	41.11
1929-31	......57.71	60.75	60.41	59.74	58.96	58.14	53.73	49.18	44.88	40.79
1939-41	....61.60	64.00	63.35	62.53	61.66	60.76	56.12	51.43	46.91	42.51
1949-51	....65.47	66.73	65.89	64.99	64.06	63.12	58.35	53.56	48.92	44.36
1955	..........66.6	67.6	....	....	....	63.9	59.1	54.3	49.6	45.1
1960	..........66.6	67.6	....	....	....	63.9	59.1	54.2	49.6	45.0
1965	..........66.8	67.7	....	....	....	64.0	59.1	54.3	49.6	45.0
1966	..........66.7	67.5	....	....	....	63.8	58.9	54.1	49.4	44.9
United Kingdom, England and Wales, Male										
1901-10	......48.53	55.68	57.00	56.92	56.49	55.90	51.81	47.31	43.01	38.86
1910-12	......51.50	57.51	58.53	....	....	57.14	53.08	48.57	44.21	....
1920-22	......55.62	60.07	60.50	....	....	58.81	54.64	50.12	45.78	....
1930-32	......58.74	62.25	62.21	61.62	60.89	60.11	55.79	51.19	46.81	42.54
1948	........66.39	68.01	67.20	66.33	65.41	64.49	59.76	54.94	50.29	45.66
1950	........66.49	67.80	66.95	66.06	65.12	64.18	59.41	54.57	49.83	45.17
1955	........67.52	68.47	67.58	66.65	65.70	64.74	59.90	55.02	50.26	45.54
1960	......68.3	69.0	68.1	67.1	66.2	65.2	60.4	55.5	50.7	46.0
1963-65	....68.30	68.90	68.00	67.00	66.10	65.10	60.30	55.40	50.60	45.90

* Prior to 1960 excluding Hawaii, and prior to 1959 excluding Alaska.

† 1900-11: data are for the ten death-registration states of 1900. 1919-21: for the 34 death-registration states of 1920.

might be another reason for the danger in being a male. But longer survival of females is noticeable even in closed and protected communities of monks and nuns, and they don't smoke.

See the fall-off in the general improvement, from 30 percent increased expectation of life at birth to 16 percent at age thirty-five and 13 percent at age fifty in the United Kingdom. In the United States the drop is even more catastrophic, from 30 percent to 11 percent to 9 percent respectively. These latter figures are the most significant, since what happens in the United States today obtains in the rest of the Western world tomorrow.

What is happening? What are the main causes of death today? Why? Study the current mortality reports and catch the trends.

30	35	40	45	50	55	60	65	70	75	80	85
34.76	31.19	27.65	24.14	20.70	17.38	14.33	11.50	9.02	6.84	5.11	3.82
34.70	30.94	27.32	23.77	20.32	16.98	13.95	11.24	8.83	6.75	5.10	3.90
37.26	33.43	29.63	25.84	22.11	18.53	15.22	12.20	9.52	7.31	5.49	4.10
36.71	32.65	28.68	24.87	21.23	17.79	14.62	11.72	9.18	7.02	5.27	4.02
38.13	33.79	29.57	25.52	21.72	18.20	14.99	12.07	9.46	7.22	5.44	4.11
39.78	35.23	30.79	26.55	22.59	18.96	15.68	12.74	10.11	7.83	5.94	4.41
40.5	35.9	31.4	27.0	23.0	19.3	15.9	12.9	10.4	8.1	6.2	5.0
40.4	35.7	31.2	26.9	22.8	19.2	15.8	12.8	10.2	7.9	6.0	4.5
40.4	35.8	31.3	27.0	22.9	19.2	15.9	12.9	10.4	8.1	6.2	4.5
40.3	35.7	31.2	26.9	22.9	19.1	15.8	12.8	10.3	8.2	6.2	4.5
34.76	30.79	26.96	23.27	19.76	16.48	13.49	10.80	8.39	6.41	4.86	3.53
35.81	....	27.74	....	20.29	....	13.78	10.99	8.53	....	....	....
37.40	....	29.19	....	21.36	....	14.36	11.36	8.75	....	....	....
38.21	33.87	29.62	25.51	21.60	17.89	14.43	11.30	8.62	6.43	4.74	3.50
41.04	36.43	31.86	27.42	23.25	19.34	15.82	12.75	10.03	7.73	5.92	4.71
40.51	35.85	31.24	26.75	22.54	18.62	15.09	12.00	9.31	7.03	5.24	3.95
40.79	36.05	31.37	26.82	22.49	18.52	14.96	11.83	9.14	6.84	5.10	3.86
41.3	36.5	31.8	27.3	22.9	18.9	15.3	12.2	19.5	7.3	5.5	4.3
41.10	36.30	31.60	27.10	22.80	18.70	15.10	12.00	9.40	7.10	5.30	4.00

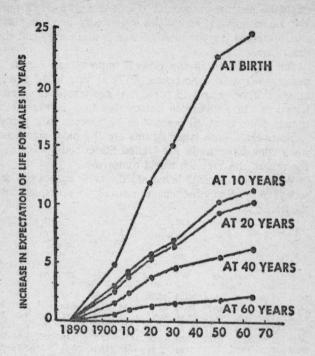

Figure 5
*Increase in Expectation of Life for Males
at Different Ages from 1881-1965*

If you live in a privileged country, and particularly if you are a man, there are two constant threats to your life. They are the more dangerous if your circumstances are such that they operate simultaneously. One is that you allow yourself to age before your time. You die sooner from what would probably have knocked you off later. The second is the running of a specific risk, that "something" (or things) in the Western way of life that you encounter that leads inexorably to the Western way of death. In Europe and North America, atherosclerosis—fatty, obstructing deposits in the arteries—is the top killer through

Figure 6
Principal Causes of Death—United States

CURRENT MORTALITY REPORT
1969 Compared with 1968 and 1964-68

Cause of Death	Death Rates Per 100,000 in 1969	1969 Death Rate as Percent of That in 1968	1964-68
All Causes	602.6	99%	98%
Major cardiovascular-renal diseases	305.7	97	95
Diseases of heart	241.7	98	94
Ischemic and related heart disease†	221.3	100	96
Cancer all forms	130.1	100	99
Respiratory system	31.0	100	104
Accidents all forms	35.7	99	102
Motor vehicle	17.3	98	101
Pneumonia and influenza	16.2	118	117
Cirrhosis of the liver	10.5	102	105
Diabetes mellitus	8.8	101	98
Suicide	7.4	96	91
War deaths	4.0	65	*
Tuberculosis	0.9	79	67

General Population of the United States—First Ten Months

All Causes	948.1	100%	101%
Major cardiovascular-renal diseases	497.5	98	98
Diseases of heart	362.5	98	99
Ischemic and related heart disease†	332.4	98	104
Cancer all forms	160.4	101	103
Accidents all forms	55.6	100	101
Motor vehicle	26.2	98	104
Pneumonia and influenza	35.5	109	113
Diabetes mellitus	18.5	99	106
Cirrhosis of the liver	15.0	106	115
Suicide	10.8	102	100
Tuberculosis	2.7	84	71

* Comparison not meaningful.
† Includes coronary heart disease.

its complications, coronary-artery disease and stroke. In the United States it is responsible for more than half the male deaths—more than all other causes of death put together: lung cancer, car accidents, Vietnam—all of them.

Apart from these, all at epidemic proportion, other dooms are looming up, like cirrhosis of the liver, increasing rapidly in the United States, as a result of alcoholism.

Figure 7
Principal Causes of Death—England and Wales

Cause of death	Average 1958-60	1966	1967	1968
Typhoid and paratyphoid fevers	....	....	2	4
Other intestinal infectious diseases	831	944	920	731
Tuberculosis, respiratory	3,043	1,810	1,580	1,456
Tuberculosis, other forms	806	508	486	635
Diphtheria	....	....	....	1
Whoopin cough	30	23	27	15
Streptococcal, sore throat and scarlet fever	18	5	7	4
Meningococcal infection	142	116	89	107
Acute poliomyelitis	1	1	1	....
Smallpox	....	....	....	....
Measles	60	81	100	51
Syphilis	507	295	264	185
Other infective and parasitic diseases	900	943	834	1,001
Malignant neoplasms:				
Stomach	14,009	13,137	12,940	2,749
Trachea, bronchus and lung	20,891	26,941	28,188	28,836
Breast	8,950	9,896	10,313	10,280
Uterus	4,041	3,924	3,854	3,971
Leukemia	2,533	2,891	2,902	3,132
Other malignant neoplasms	46,498	50,963	52,128	53,583
Diabetes mellitus	3,347	4,295	4,239	4,616
Ischemic heart disease	109,064	130,113	129,204	138,617
Cerebrovascular disease	74,615	77,540	76,988	80,352
Acute bronchitis and bronchiolitis	3,091	2,753	2,292	2,792
Influenza	3,760	3,644	883	4,652
Pneumonia	25,119	35,307	32,231	41,027
Bronchitis (other than acute)	25,332	29,313	25,946	29,864
Emphysema and asthma	2,333	3,289	3,000	2,902
Ulcer of stomach and duodenum ..	4,338	3,752	3,561	3,832
Gastritis and duodenitis	83	66	77	73
Nephritis and nephrosis	3,567	2,320	2,218	2,468
Hyperplasia of prostate	3,530	2,004	1,804	1,580
Complications of pregnancy, childbirth and puerperium	287	214	173	200
Congenital anomalies	5,047	4,810	4,693	4,752
All other diseases	131,677	121,401	117,170	119,543
Motor vehicle accidents	5,983	7,383	7,168	6,349
Accidental poisoning by drugs and medicaments	167	369	407	399
Accidental poisoning by other solid and liquid substances	26	40	37	43
Accidental poisoning by gases and vapours	785	733	569	522
Suicide and self-inflicted injury	5,135	4,929	4,668	4,584
All other accidents, poisonings and violence	10,407	10,637	10,553	10,846
Total All causes	526,921	557,390	542,516	576,754

In British mental hospitals three times as many patients are being admitted for alcoholic psychosis as ten years ago. Diabetes is inching up, too, especially the diet-dependent type. In a recent study in Bedford, England, 50 percent of women of fifty were found to be prediabetic, with the concomitant dangers of blood-vessel troubles in the legs, eyes, heart, brain, and kidneys. Heroin is top teen-age killer in New York. All of these are lethal results of the way we choose to live: you don't have to choose it.

Man has always found ways of killing himself prematurely, for dietary, social, religious, or political causes. Death from old age alone was and is comparatively rare. The common cause of death is accident, in which term is included disease. But whatever the illness, accident, or degenerative condition that strikes the fatal blow, the victims it is most likely to catch up with are the old. It is the worn part that cracks up, the aging tissue that lacks resistance. Whatever causes aging, it is nothing as simple as time. It depends on the passing, expenditure, accumulation, or happening of something other than mere years; unlike the way the "life" of an aircraft can be calculated in flying hours, or the "life" of a bottle of whiskey can be determined by the number of jiggers taken out. We don't know what the "something" is for us.

The central problem of our time and place and culture is the development of malignant aging among some of us.

Malignant aging means that physical changes normally associated with middle age and senescence come on early among some people, so that the changes may be well advanced by the twenties and thirties. In their next two decades such people will be as vulnerable to disease or disaster—particularly of certain kinds—as others are likely to be in their seventies and eighties.

Paradoxically, malignant aging is often part of what looks like the beginning of a success story: it never reaches the happy ending. The victim is of the type with drive and energy; he is likely to have been popular and made a name for himself at college in sports as well as in academic subjects; he might have been a team captain. He marries early, works hard, and takes on responsibility. He is restless and active, and his mood swings between anxiety and boredom, but he cannot spare time for exercise or relaxation. His only recreation is eating and drinking. He drives fast. He has business lunches and work to take home on weekends.

Success is in sight for him early, but he may die before he can reach out to grasp it. If you are moderately prosperous and on the way up, and live in a modern city, you could be the type: like Sam or Wally. If you are a woman with the same dynamic drive you run something of the same risk but much less dangerously.

If aging were something that started with retirement, or even at a set age like thirty-five, malignant aging could not occur. But life is a one-way journey, like a nonstop train trip on a single track. Aging is a continuous process all the way—it may be retarded or accelerated but it is always going on.

Sir Robert Platt, professor of medicine at the University of Manchester, in his presidential address to the Royal Society of Medicine, pointed out that we are all aging from the fertilization of the ovum onward. Aging in the early years includes maturing, developing resistance to disease, and the ability to avoid accidents. The years of greatest fitness, when death in the next twelve months is least likely, are those from ten to twelve. You are never so safe again.

Basic intelligence is at a maximum at about eighteen years, although learning and experience continue and compensate for the gradual falling off. The peak age for creativity averages thirty-five, with painters touching the top at twenty-two, poets at thirty, novelists at forty-five, and millionaires at fifty. The height of athletic prowess usually runs from twenty to twenty-five, while fertility is greatest for men at twenty-five to thirty and for women several years earlier. Because of better nutrition, people nowadays grow taller and attain their full physical stature two or three years younger than a century ago. Girls begin to menstruate this much earlier than in Jane Austen's time, too. But such "improvements" may be associated with earlier aging, as we shall see.

The different parts of body and mind develop and

mature at different rates, and these rates vary with each individual. One boy of fourteen may look and sound like a grown man, while another, just as normal, may have the voice and physique of a child. One may be mature mentally but immature in his emotions, another may be sexually adult before the rest.

As with maturing, similarly with the gradual degenerative changes we understand as aging. One aspect or organ may be affected sooner than another, and in one person sooner than in another. One man may be bald at twenty-five, one woman gray at thirty. These are obvious changes, but of little significance for health, and largely independent of experience or environment—though you may go gray sooner from worry. But other parts, such as the blood vessels or kidneys, may also age sooner in one person than in another, and these can matter vitally. Impaired functioning of one organ or system may affect others, and the results are far-reaching when, for instance, the blood vessels to certain glands begin to fail.

If an important organ receives an insult from accident, bacterial attack, chronic strain, or irritation, this may either hasten the aging process or prove too much for a part already suffering age changes. For instance, the special factors which lead prematurely to coronary thrombosis are superimposed on that arterial degeneration that occurs inevitably, and this also seems to be influenced powerfully by the diet, etc.

Aging starts sooner than you think. The eyes begin gradually to lose their power of accommodation from about age eight; the acuity of hearing high notes falls off infinitesimally also. It is from about age twenty-five that more important changes, just then beginning, may become detectable. The British United Provident Association (BUPA), the largest private medical-insurance company in the country, recommends regular checkups from twenty-five onward. By this age there are straws in the wind to indicate where evasive action or vigorous reaction is needed for survival.

The fatty changes in the walls of the arteries that spell atherosclerosis and early death for thousands have been found in apparently fit young servicemen in their teens and early twenties in Vietnam. Dr. Lawrence Lamb, professor of cardiology at Baylor University in Texas, found deposits in the arteries of 77 percent of Americans killed in Korea —average age twenty-two. Some hearts were already scarred by disease at thirty. Age changes cannot be altogether prevented, but they need not be hastened, and in atherosclerosis at least, eating habits affect its progress. Sometimes compensatory developments may be induced. For instance, small, reserve blood vessels supplying the heart can be encouraged to open up and take over from others which have silted up, and physical exercise may make a forty-year-old muscular system in one man operate more efficiently than another's at twenty. Muscle strength, measured by the grip on a dynamometer, usually falls off noticeably at around thirty, yet Stan Matthews, the British footballer, and tennis players Cochet and Borotra played at international standard in their fifties.

The skin characteristically becomes thinner and loses its elasticity with age. Pinch up a little on the back of your hand and notice how long it takes to go flat compared with a pinch on your abdomen or some other part not exposed. It does not matter if the skin on your hands is showing signs of wear, but it is an indication that changes may be going on elsewhere in your body, and that *these* changes may be affected by what you do or how you live. The devastating effects of tropical sun on a woman's complexion, or of detergents and domestic work on her hands, show too the influence of a person's habits on his rate of aging.

Other normal concomitants of growing older, which could be serious if allowed to get out of hand, include a gradual rise in the blood pressure; a falling off in the blood flow through the kidneys so that poisonous waste products accumulate; and reduced efficiency in using carbohydrates, so that diabetes may threaten. Food is converted into protein—flesh—in the young, but to fat in the middle-aged. Sexual activity often, but not inevitably, diminishes with increased age. There has been an attractive—for men—theory current for about three thousand years that sex with a young, pretty woman will rejuvenate a man. As a new interest in his life it could well do something good for his psyche, but active sex glands do not, in fact, extend a man's life. Monkey glands and sex hormones did nothing for C. E. Brown-Séquard and those who followed him, except to give them short-lived hope.

Professor Tanner, growth expert at the Institute of Child Development in London, believes that a series of signals from the cortex, the thinking part of the brain, spark off the bodily changes of puberty, when a child matures to adulthood. The same process occurs with the changes of degeneration. Professor F. C. Bartlett and his colleagues in Cambridge, England, have found that the psychological changes of aging precede the physical ones. Psychological senescence is noticeable in most of us in the mid-twenties—when we steady down—and is usually well advanced by forty. It includes firm convictions—"knowing your own mind"—a dogmatic attitude, a falling off in the appetite for adventure and change for their own sake, reliability and predictability, a growing resistance to new ideas, especially if these involve learning, and caution and conventionality. One takes oneself seriously, and sex becomes a domestic habit like brushing the teeth.

At the opposite pole are a little lunacy, a sense of the ridiculous, imagination and impulsiveness, unlikely enthusiasms, and what might be called a poor work record. To ward off mental aging it seems that a change of major intellectual interest, in most cases in one's work, is necessary at least every ten or twelve years.

The overriding effect of the outlook and state of mind shows up in the case of widows and widowers in the younger age groups. The premature death rate for these people is higher than for the married or the single, right across the board—from heart disease, cancer, accidents, infections—all causes. On the other side of the coin are those whose youthful minds and imaginations kept their bodies going long past the normal span, even without any particular care for their health—men such as Maugham, Bertrand Russell, Churchill, and Shaw; or in earlier times, Michelangelo and Verdi.

Apart from growing middle-aged, mind first, before it is time, you can throw the best part of your life into the ashcan by running specific risks, usually by some excess, as it's always been. Henry II of England died of a surfeit of lampreys (a nasty kind of fish); Henry VIII from a surfeit of wives; and the Black Prince from a surfeit of battles. Our excesses today include eating, so that chronic overnutrition is by far the commonest malnutrition in the West; drinking; drugging; smoking cigarettes; and sitting —in cars, offices, cinemas, or while watching TV. Fast, aggressive driving holds today the same dashing and romantic appeal as did the Crusades and is more dangerous. We subject ourselves to psychosomatic (psychosomatic: damaging the body through the mind) stresses as never before by entering the rat race. Businessmen live by the sword and no one knows who will be cut down next. And there's no letup between battles, as used to occur in the days of the visible sword.

An unhealthy environment, like Belsen, the Congo basin, or a Neapolitan slum, means that more people die younger: prematurely. A large part of your personal environment is up to you. The intense pollution of the atmosphere you breathe if you smoke a cigarette has been shown, by testing the rise of carbon monoxide in the blood, to be far more severe than exposure to all the car exhaust fumes during the evening exodus from London or New York. The food factor is another that is personal to you: it is your mouth that is the sole port of entry for excessive or unsuitable food. Consider McCay of Cornell and his rats. He found that rats that were slightly underfed in calories though not in quality of diet matured more slowly but regularly lived twice as long as those who were given all they needed all their lives. The underfed rats, when middle-aged, also had all the appearance and sprightliness of youth. This is why it does not seem a matter for much self-congratulation that by bigger food supplies we have enabled ourselves to mature sooner than our grandparents did. In another set of experiments, adult mice who fasted for two days each week had their life span increased by 60 percent—some hint that restraint in food intake may be beneficial, even after maturity.

The new epidemics of our day are every bit as deadly as the Black Death of seven centuries ago. The difference is that then they had no idea how to avoid the disaster, whereas now we have the information, if we care to put it into practice. For instance, the chances of dropping dead from a coronary or choking your life out with lung cancer before your allotted time are, we know, far greater if you smoke cigarettes. It is significant that those in a position to see the evidence with their own eyes, the doctors, are pulling out of danger themselves. Four fifths of American doctors and seven tenths of British doctors are among those interesting deviates from conventional behavior—people who don't smoke. The lung cancer death rate for doctors in Britain has gone down by a third, while for the rest of the population it has risen by a quarter.

The message that shines through is that if we study the facts, then use sense and self-control, we stand a good chance of not dying young.

There are two absurd anomalies in the way we organize our health affairs in the West today. It would be ludicrous, if it were not so sad, to think of all the money, publicity, and high skill spent on transplants—temporary patch-ups of already worn frames—and so little on teaching men to live so that their own hearts, arteries, and other organs can serve them through a reasonable span. Secondly, it seems crazy to spend a third to a half of one's potential life in growing, learning, and preparing for one's big part, and then to allow oneself to be hustled off the stage partway through the performance—as may happen if one still chooses to ignore the evidence, the way Sam did, and Wally, and Caroline and Philip.

2

What Can Kill You;
What Can't

There's no need to go into a spin if you sneeze, nor make notes for your obituary if you find you have a bunion. Neither is a killing disease. If you feel headachy and feverish, don't panic. It's unlikely in this day, age, and place that you have picked up a fatal dose of the bubonic plague or even smallpox, and however naughty you've been the chances are negligible that you'll die of VD. You can be in agony with an aching molar, or prostrate in a darkened room with migraine, feeling like death, and yet be nowhere near it.

Your memory may fail, but if your more vital functions continue, so will you. You may be crippled with arthritis, blind, or deaf and still survive. Doris Hart won the highest tennis honors at Wimbledon despite a polio-crippled leg. Franklin D. could lead a nation from a wheelchair, until . . .

A minimal leak in an artery to the brain can spell *curtains* for you as it did for him. If your heart stalls or you don't draw a breath in for four minutes, you're done for immediately. Any impairment of the pumping, oxygenating, fueling, or waste-disposal systems or their computerized controls in the brain is potentially deadly. These are the risk areas. Let's look at them for a moment.

The pumping system: You know that if you get a bullet in your heart, that's it. A coronary clot can also produce instant death. It is heart disease or heart disaster that finishes more of us than anything else. Cardiovascular-renal disorders (heart, arteries, kidneys) account for 52 percent of American deaths, 47 percent of British. If you want to go on, you must give your heart a chance to do the same, but the "with-it" way of life may hinder this.

Fuel pipes: You know that if you slash an artery and all your blood runs out you'll die. The pumping system is pointless without serviceable pipelines—arteries that can cope with a pulsing flow of nutrients and oxygen-bearing hemoglobin to the tissues. Your number is up—just as surely as from that slash—if your arteries are clogged by greasy atherosclerosis, blocked by clotting of the blood in them (thrombosis) or by detached fragments from a clot elsewhere (embolism), or if they are stiff and subject to cracking and leakage as in arteriosclerosis. A stroke is the cracking or clotting of the blood of an artery in the brain: it finished FDR and continues to strike down others who choose the Western way of life.

A weak place in an artery wall, like a blister in a rubber tube, is a constant threat to life if it involves a main vessel or one in the brain. This condition is known as an aneurysm, and the commonest type is produced by the same habits of living as lead to arteriosclerosis.

Your arteriovenous system of fuel pipes needs to be kept in prime order, for it is an old medical saw that a man is as old as his arteries. What are you doing about yours?

Hypertension means that the blood pressure in the arteries is raised above what the body is built to stand. It kills by the strains it imposes on the heart, which has to pump against enormous resistance, or on the arteries, which may give way to the pressure, because of the destruction of the delicate selection and filtration apparatus of the kidneys. If you are an American, hypertension is a very major threat to your celebrating your golden anniversary. But you can do something to save the situation, especially now.

Oxygenating system: This includes the lungs and the airways leading into them: the windpipe, the bronchi, and the smaller tubes, or bronchioles, which end in the myriad air sacs where the gaseous exchanges actually take place. Oxygen is absorbed into the bloodstream, and waste carbon dioxide released to be disposed of when you breathe out. Oxygen is vital for the slow chemical combustion processes that are the essence of life, underlying your thinking, moving, speaking, digesting, and reproducing. It is continuously required. The brain cannot survive five minutes without oxygen, and the heart dies in eight, while less vital parts may take a little longer before they go.

You know that if you gulp in a chunk of meat the wrong way and it blocks the entrance to your lungs you're a goner. The end result is the same if your lungs are out of service for any other reason. Lung diseases that are likely to kill you quite slowly are cancer and chronic bronchitis, or emphysema. These are common exit signs in Britain, and serious threats in the United States. Rare these days, but acting through the same system, is tuberculosis: it killed the poet Keats and most of the Brontë family, young. It was lung cancer that choked George VI to death in our century, early in the epidemic.

Quick-acting killers in the oxygenating system include pneumonia, influenza pneumonia, and acute bronchitis— more likely to prove lethal if they come on top of some other trouble. These and the long-term lung diseases are disasters that, in most cases, you can avoid.

The fueling system: Comprises the gullet, the stomach, the intestines, and the rectum, plus various offshoots and glands. It doesn't cause death within the hour if some parts are injured or diseased. But, like an airplane, sooner or later you'll crash if your fueling system develops a fault. A common cause of trouble is a peptic ulcer: either in the stomach (gastric ulcer) or in the two-inch stretch of intestine that leads out of it (duodenal ulcer). A sudden death can occur from such a complication as perforation, when the ulcer eats right through the stomach wall. Cancers of the stomach and the lower end of the digestive tract, the colon and rectum, can also prove fatal if not caught in the bud.

The liver is closely associated with the food tract. It is through the liver that unprocessed chyle from the collecting vessels around the intestines is converted into usable form, either for immediate combustion or to keep in storage. The liver holds a key place in your body's functioning. It is a seething, multipurpose chemical plant, running at a higher temperature than any other part of the body and situated under the ribs on the right—in a secluded yet central position, like a penthouse on Fifth Avenue or London's Park Lane. One important function of the liver is the detoxification of poisons, both those released by the body's own chemistry and those from outside. Its efficient working is a must for your survival.

Infectious hepatitis is the commonest acute disorder of the liver, and it is causing some worrying deaths among really young adults. This needs watching. Cirrhosis of the liver is, however, a much commoner cause of death, and is taking a seriously increasing toll in the United States. It is an eminently avoidable disease.

Another organ associated wtih the digestive system is the pancreas. It provides an enzyme necessary for digesting protein, and it also produces insulin. A lack of insulin produces diabetes—another major cause of death today. Again, habits—in this case, dietary—may predispose one to the development of the disease.

The top-risk areas are your heart and arteries, your lungs, and your digestive system: not your big toe, your ear, or your emotions.

This is reflected in the order of today's major causes of death:

1. Diseases of the heart and arteries, 52 percent.
2. Cancer, including lung, breast, and stomach, 22 percent.
3. Accident, 6 percent.
4. Pneumonia and influenza, 2 percent.

5. Cirrhosis of the liver, 1.5 percent (United States only).
6. Diabetes, 1.5 percent.

Cancer and accidents are in a special category: they can kill you by wrecking any part of the body. At first, a group of cancer cells, especially if these cells are in some organ that is not in constant use, such as the breast or the prostate gland, are no threat to life; if they are cut out or destroyed by radiation at this stage there is no harm done. But if some from the gang of wild, pathological cells get loose in the bloodstream or in that other system of vessels, the lymphatics, they may be carried to some vital part, often the lungs, liver, or control area of the brain. It is because of this that an early-warning system is important for cancer. Some cancers, like lung cancer, may be avoidable, but this does not apply to the majority of them.

To keep it "all systems go" for a reasonable life span you need to care for your body at least as well as for your car. You need to get it inspected periodically and examined for minor faults that might cause trouble later and for signs of wear or damage. For a car it is called servicing; for a human body, screening. Any small abnormalities should be dealt with promptly, even if they don't seem too important in themselves. You can see why when you think about accidents.

You can smash yourself up in a car and even more completely on a motorbike. You can electrocute yourself, get in the way of a train, or drop five hundred feet from a cliff. These may seem pretty straightforward ways of getting rubbed out, and certainly there's not much you can do if the aircraft that you are traveling in is hijacked or flies bang into a mountain. But the likelihood of home, work, or road accidents is multiplied many times over if your mood is angry, suicidal, anxious, or plain bored; if you are alcoholic, tired, or otherwise dopey; if you didn't have your eyes checked and you need new glasses; if you are taking antihistamine pills for hay fever, etc; if you have a pain or an epileptic fit; if you are cooking up a fever, have a heartache (either emotion-based or cardiac) or kidney colic . . .

Or think of it another way. You have a minor accident on the road—take a spill off your bicycle and cut your leg. So what? So too bad, if the varicose vein you were going to have operated on is injured and you lose three pints of blood. It is a mistake to think an accident is only what it seems. Keeping your body in "impeccable condition," as the automobile salesmen put it, may help you to avoid an accidental death as much as any other means of prevention. But there are still some things which are complete nonworries; such things as baldness, flat feet, or acne may annoy, but they certainly won't kill you. Even among the World Health Organization's listed causes of death there are a good many that are no real threat to you.

MINIMAL RISKS

Combing through the medical and mortality statistics for 250 countries, put out annually by the United Nations and WHO, you get an idea of which diseases are comparatively likely to kill you young, and which are not. For instance, if you live in the West and you are between twenty-five and fifty-five years of age the chances are less than one in 100,000 of your dying—directly—from one of these conditions:

Syphilis, gonorrhea—forms of VD.

Typhoid, paratyphoid, salmonella, cholera, brucellosis, dysentery—diarrheal illnesses.

Strep throat, scarlet fever, erysipelas—streptococcal infections.

Measles, yellow fever, diphtheria, whooping cough, plague, leprosy, tetanus, polio, rabies, typhus, malaria, tropical parasites—killers of other times, other places.

Goiter, thyrotoxicosis—thyroid-gland disorders.

Inflammation of the eye, cataract, glaucoma—eye diseases.

Otitis media, rheumatic fever, infections of the nose, throat, and sinuses, pleurisy, bone infection—bacterial diseases now beaten by antibiotics.

Gastritis, appendicitis, acute kidney disease.

Abortion, whether septic or uncomplicated.

Arthritis, rheumatism (except for rheumatic heart disease).

Yet all of these are listed as causes of death for some.

If you are a woman in the West you are unlikely to die from duodenal ulcer, drowning, fire, or accidents with machinery—though it's quite in the cards if you are a man. A woman doesn't run a significant risk of developing a cancer of the larynx, nor—obviously—of the prostate, just as a man can't develop a uterine cancer, and won't expect to get a cancer of the breast.

You are safer in Britain than in the United States from homicide, lethal gall-bladder trouble, cirrhosis, diabetes, and high blood pressure, but you cannot discount them on either side of the Atlantic. Similarly, in the United States, you run less risk of chronic bronchitis, emphysema, and anemia.

WHAT COULD KILL YOU?

Let's take a look at those conditions that hold a substantial risk for someone of your age.

Unless otherwise stated, death rates per 100,000 are given, for those aged forty-five to fifty-four years. Of course, the illness would have been coming on before the death, and in most cases the death rates for ages thirty-five to forty-four are about half those for forty-five to fifty-four.

Cast your eyes down the list, and pay particular attention to conditions that caught up with your friends, your kind of people. Take account, even more, where a relative

	United States		United Kingdom		Sweden	
	Men	Women	Men	Women	Men	Women
TB of the Lung	8.9	2.5	5.5	2.7	—	—
Cancers						
Mouth and pharynx (back of throat)	8.8	2.7	3.2	1.7	—	—
Gullet	5.6	1.8	4.9	2.4	—	—
Stomach	9.1	4.8	21.1	9.5	—	—
(ages 35–44)	2.5	1.6	4.0	2.6	—	—
Intestine	12.7	14.2	11.1	14.0	—	—
(ages 35–44)	3.3	4.2	3.4	4.5	—	—
Rectum	5.2	4.0	7.4	6.5	—	—
Larynx	3.4	.7	1.7	.5	—	—
Lung	61.4	16.1	83.3	21.8	20.5	6.1
(Cigarette advertising is banned in Sweden)						
(ages 35–44)	14.0	5.0	14.0	5.0	—	—
Breast	.3	52.6	.3	58.2	—	—
Cervix		14.7		19.9	—	—
(ages 35–44)		8.0		8.0	—	—
Womb		5.3		4.3	—	—
Prostate	2.4		1.6		—	—
Skin	4.5	2.7	2.1	2.0	—	—
Bone	1.5	1.5	1.5	1.5	—	—
Leukemia (blood cancer)	6.8	4.9	4.9	3.6	—	—
Diabetes	12.5	12.2	3.4	2.5	—	—
Allergic disorders (such as asthma)	6.5	6.5	6.5	6.5	—	—
Psychological disorders						
Psychosis	1.9	—	—	—	—	—
Psychoneurosis	5.9	2.1	—	—	—	—

(Difficult to define: differences in figures are probably an artificial effect of different diagnostic criteria in the two countries.)

Suicide

(The ultimate in psychological upset, and easier to define. It is too important a cause of death to ignore. Men outnumber women at all ages. It seems worse where the standard of living is highest, e.g., in the United States compared with the United Kingdom. Compare Sweden, which has the most in peace and prosperity.)

	United States		United Kingdom		Sweden	
(ages 45–54)	27.5	12.1	16.8	12.9	55.6	20.8
(ages 35–44)	22.9	10.7	13.8	8.7	43.5	15.2
(ages 25–34)	17.2	7.6	11.5	5.3		
Stroke	46.2	41.0	41.4	40.6	27.2	23.3
(ages 35–44)	15.0	15.0	12.0	12.0		
Epilepsy	About 1.5 all classes					
Rheumatic heart disease	11.2	12.5	13.4	17.9	—	—
Arteriosclerotic and degenerative heart disease (includes coronary disease)						
All ages	383.7	251.9	349.1	269.6	—	—
45–54	351.8	80.0	244.0	41.6	133.7	25.4
35–44	93.0	19.8	64.5	10.0	—	—

	United States Men	United States Women	United Kingdom Men	United Kingdom Women	Sweden Men	Sweden Women
Other heart diseases	15.9	7.8	7.3	4.4	—	—
High blood pressure (with heart trouble)	19.0	14.0	5.2	3.3	5.5	1.7
Diseases of arteries	9.0	4.3	6.9	3.0	—	—
(These more often cause death through stroke or heart disease.)						
Lobar pneumonia	4.8	1.9	3.6	1.9	—	—
Bronchopneumonia (half these figures for ages 35–44)	9.8	4.6	8.7	6.7	—	—
Acute bronchitis	—	—	1.3	—	—	—
Chronic bronchitis	2.5	1.0	28.3	8.6	2.3	.6
Stomach ulcer	3.9	1.5	2.7	1.0	—	—
Duodenal ulcer	3.4	1.1	2.2	.9	—	—
Gastroenteritis	2.2	1.9	1.6	2.0	—	—
Cirrhosis	45.2	25.0	3.8	3.8	14.9	5.9
Gall bladder disease (worse in older ages in United Kingdom)	1.0	1.2	—	—	—	—
Chronic nephritis (kidney disease)	7.4	5.1	6.2	3.7	—	—
Kidney infections	2.5	3.8	1.0	1.8	—	—
Car crashes						
ages 15–24	76.3	21.3	40.7	9.4	32.4	10.5
ages 25–34	50.8	13.1	18.5	4.1	—	—
ages 35–44	36.7	12.4	14.3	4.0	—	—
ages 45–54	37.9	14.4	16.8	6.4	—	—
Other transport accidents	6.1	.6	2.3	.4	—	—
Accidental poisoning	4.5	1.4	3.8	3.6	—	—
Falls	9.1	2.9	4.2	1.4	—	—
Machinery accidents	3.3	—	1.6	—	—	—
Fire	5.5	2.7	1.1	—	—	—
Drowning	3.3	—	1.6	—	—	—
Homicide	13.1	3.6	—	—	—	—
Anemia	1.8	1.7	2.4	4.2	—	—
and—for the record—						
Senility (all ages)	.7	1.1	4.7	10.5	—	—

was affected. This is not meant to give you the jitters, but to enable you to take the most effective evasive action that's most appropriate for a man or woman like you.

Some models of automobile and aircraft are prone to develop a particular fault because of weak points in their design. Some people are liable to particular health troubles because of their constitution. In calculating your best course of action for survival consider the sort of person you are.

What you are like—plump, prosperous, and expansive,

or long, lean, lanky, and intellectual, to mention two extreme types—depends upon your heredity and your environment interacting. Your heredity is the legacy your parents gave you before you were born. At the moment of conception a kind of genetic blueprint of your potentialities and possible weaknesses is laid down, and as you develop from an ovum this is copied into every cell of your body, indelibly.

The genes which are in control come half from one parent and half from the other. Nothing can alter them or erase the messages they give out. Some are quick-acting, for instance those that determine the color of your eyes. The influence of others may not show until comparatively late in life, like the genes that make for baldness, which can operate only when the male sex hormones reach a certain level; or those which induce high blood pressure, or more specific diseases, like Huntington's chorea.

Operating alongside the forces of heredity, maybe in conjunction with them or maybe against them, are the effects of environment. Environment means everything outside you that impinges on you. Your mother's womb was your earliest environment. Since then, your upbringing in matters of behavior and morals, the training of your tastes in food, your emotional life and stresses, medical care, school experience, and work—all have been environmental factors exerting an influence on your constitution.

No matter how marvelous your hereditary possibilities, your environment can wreck them. For instance, you might have the potential for being a fine musician but never have the opportunity to learn an instrument; you might have the legs and lung capacity to be a miler, but spoil your chances by becoming a chain smoker. On the other hand, a very good heredity can sometimes carry a man to the top, in spite of heavy environmental odds against him. Abraham Lincoln was one such man, Lord Nuffield, the car magnate, another, while in show business the Cinderella story is almost the norm.

Conversely, a helpful environment can do a great deal to compensate for a crippling heredity. A child with spina bifida used invariably to die young or drag out a useless wheelchair existence into adulthood. There is still no cure, but if a child so afflicted gets into a special school (the optimum environment for someone with his condition), he can learn to walk with braces, manage his disabilities independently, and develop his talents for earning a living in the outside world.

What you could be on your genetic endowment alone is called your *genotype*. Your *phenotype*, much the same as your constitution, is what you actually are—the product of your genotype and your environment; your potentialities and possibilities in a blend.

The value of knowing something of your heredity is that you can then manipulate your environment to suit it. For instance, if several members of your family have had gout, it would be wise not to take up drinking as a serious pastime nor acquire a particular taste for purine-containing foodstuffs, like sardines and sweetbreads. If emphysema or bronchitis has been a frequent trouble among your relatives you would be sticking your neck out if you took a job where the atmosphere was dusty, or if you smoked.

In some conditions heredity plays a clear-cut role. Hemophilia, for instance, depends entirely of the genes, and all you can do to mitigate its effects is to avoid accidents, and to arrange for prompt treatment when bleeding does occur; or, prophylactically speaking, to take all precautions when something like having a tooth out is planned.

In most cases, however, what is inherited is merely a susceptibility to a disease or disability. For example, consider rheumatic fever: this is an illness that starts with a streptococcal infection in the throat and goes on to involve the joints, and sometimes, more seriously and permanently, the valves of the heart. A strep sore throat is commonplace: you are sure to have had some. But only a small proportion develop into rheumatic fever. Poverty, with poor housing, is one predisposing factor, but another is hereditary susceptibility. There is ten times the likelihood of developing rheumatic fever if a first-degree relative has had it.

It is rather the same with peptic ulcers. In a recent study in Northwest London it was found that fathers, mothers, brothers, and sisters of patients with gastric or duodenal ulcers had ulcers themselves twice as frequently as members of the general population in the area. Among the brothers of patients aged thirty-five plus, for instance, fifty-four had ulcers when only twenty-three would have been expected—a significant difference by any standard. It could hardly be argued that brothers of this age, each living in a different home with a different wife to cook for him, all had the same ulcer-making diet. Nor did they all do the same kind of work. A Danish study covered ulcers in the two types of twins: identical, with carbon-copy genetic equipment, and fraternal, no more alike genetically than other brothers and sisters. This study too, showed that heredity influences the development of ulcers. If one twin had an ulcer the other was far more likely to get one also if he was genetically identical.

Once you have been warned by someone else in your family getting an ulcer, you can organize your living and eating habits in order to sidestep this particular trouble.

It seems highly probable that a genetic factor is involved in the development of diabetes mellitus, but only in producing a tendency toward it. Only half of the identical twins of diabetics—with identical genes—develop the disease, so it cannot be entirely hereditary. Yet the relatives of diabetics are more likely than the population at large to develop this disorder, at the rate of one in fifteen instead of one or two per hundred. This is another situation in which your relatives provide you with an early-warning system—particularly valuable since there are a number of precipitating factors which you can aim to avoid, from obesity to car crashes to certain drugs used in medicine.

High blood pressure, a major factor today in premature death from coronary disease, stroke, and also kidney disease, is strongly influenced by heredity. The brothers and sisters of any patient going to a doctor for high blood pressure are eight times as likely as other people to have high blood pressure themselves. Sir Robert Platt says:

". . . by a carefully designed system of breeding (which is most unlikely to be adopted) essential hypertension as a common and important cause of death in middle age, could be eliminated in a few generations." By "middle age" he meant thirty-five to fifty-nine years. If both your parents have had high blood pressure the chances are about 45 percent for you, and if one parent only was affected, 30 percent. Hypertension is another condition in which a hint of the possible danger can be helpful in avoiding it, or in having treatment at a stage when it is worthwhile.

Thyroid disorders, which can have a devastating effect on the heart if untreated, also run in families. Pernicious anemia, rheumatoid arthritis, and schizophrenia also fall into the category of disorders for which there may be a hereditary disposition.

Another interesting facet of heredity and the propensity to certain diseases is the association with blood groups. For example, if you are group O you are 40 percent likelier to develop a duodenal ulcer than those of other groups. An advantage of belonging to this group, however, is that its members stand the least chance of developing a thrombosis—a reassuring thought for those taking the pill. People of blood group A run an above-average risk of developing cancer of the stomach, a condition that is curable if caught in time.

Cancer remains one of the most baffling of human afflictions. While there is no proof that heredity is directly responsible for any of the common types, it does seem that cancer of certain organs runs in some families, for instance, an uncommon type of cancer of the intestine. You may stand slightly more chance of getting a particular type of cancer if some of your relatives have had it, but if this puts you on the *qui vive* it may save your life. A cancer that has been completely removed doesn't start up again. Sometimes, of course, a type of cancer may appear to run in a family merely because several members have been exposed to the same industrial risk, or have the same habit—for instance, smoking.

An allergic tendency, which may manifest itself in

various sensitivity reactions, from hay fever to hives to asthma, is definitely hereditary. The inheritance is of a tendency to allergy in general, not to any particular disease. For instance, a mother with asthma may produce a baby with allergic eczema. There are precautionary measures that anyone with an allergic tendency should take—for instance, an avoidance of dusts, pollens, molds, and skin irritants.

But beyond all doubt the commonest and most far-reaching and serious condition for health that anyone can inherit is the male sex. It has been estimated that some 170 male zygotes are conceived to every 100 female. Something happens along the production line to redress the balance. By birth, the difference is a negligible 106 male to 100 female. Many more miscarriages turn out to have been potential boys than girls, but there must also be a big male wastage earlier on.

Boy babies stand up to the rigors of birth less well than girls. More of them have congenital defects of all kinds except congenitally dislocated hip and spina bifida. They are virtually the only victims of the sex-linked inherited diseases: progressive muscular dystrophy is one that is invariably fatal; hemophilia makes survival a chancy affair; while color blindness is a disease that doesn't matter—until one mistakes a traffic signal.

The disparity of risk diminishes a little during the mid-years of childhood, but from age fifteen right through to fifty-five, mortality rates for males considerably exceed those for the women. At forty to fifty they stand more than four times the chance of dying from a coronary attack or lung cancer; three times as many men as women die in car crashes, and from chronic bronchitis, pneumonia, ulcers, and tuberculosis; twice as many drop out permanently because of stomach cancer, arterial disease, cirrhosis, and suicide; while it is only to be expected that men run much more risk than women from accidents of all sorts and from murder—which is no accident.

Part of the high male mortality rate may be due to the way they live—working with machines, exposure to the elements—but some at least is due to their inherent weakness. The Y chromosome, that which confers masculinity, is a stunted object compared with the female X chromosomes. Besides, there is only one of it, compared with the feminine double X.

Constitution is the health aspect of your phenotype. There are three basic constitutional types, and what you are will be a mix of them all, but with a heavier loading of one or another component.

One constitutional type is the *endomorph:* smooth-skinned, rounded, and soft, with a relatively large, long trunk and small hands and feet. He has fine hair and a tendency to premature baldness, the kind that starts at the crown. The endo is sociable, sympathetic, and deservedly popular and often in the acting and singing professions. This type has a propensity to self-indulgence, which, coupled with a tendency to sink into depression, can lead to overeating and obesity, overdrinking and alcoholism, or taking drugs with the dangers attendant on that. Gall bladder trouble is common in this type.

The *mesomorph* is square, hard, rugged, and keen on sport—at least in his college days. He has massive bones and muscles, and the female of the type bears children with particular ease and efficiency. The meso's skin tans richly and soon. He has springy hair, but he too may go bald, usually from the front. This type is characteristically full of drive and aggression: he's the one that gets there —if something doesn't get him first.

The third type is the *ectomorph:* linear, fragile-looking with small, delicate bones and a triangular face, thin, palish skin and abundant hair, even in old age. He or she is surprisingly tough, and puts away—amazingly—great platefuls of meat. He often has great imagination, but little power for stirring other people. The ectomorphic constitution is unexpectedly durable—think of Bertrand Russell, at ninety, demonstrating like a student. These people are particularly resistant to cancers.

Your constitutional type has a bearing on the way you should live. For example, if you are predominantly mesomorphic, you will need, more than most, plenty of exercise and mental unwinding for your survival. Since yours is the type to rise to the top in today's world, it is of today's epidemic diseases that you must beware. If you are more of an endomorph, it is moderation you need, in eating, drinking, and other comfort habits, and you must guard against depression. You are built to run on a fuel containing a large proportion of fruit and vegetables. The life-shortening dangers of obesity should concern you and the mesomorph. As an ectomorph, you will thrive on regular, protein-rich meals, and walking, rather than organized forms of exercise.

It was Dr. Wilfrid Sheldon of Harvard who first studied scientifically the morphological classification of human beings as a botanist studies plants. He has pointed the way for others to follow in correlating consitutional types and susceptibility to disease; while a doctor who has grown wise in his practice comes to know automatically that this patient probably has duodenal ulcer, or that another is a candidate for high blood pressure. If you don't want to die young you must consider not only the killers that are general, but particularly the pitfalls for someone like you. Outwitting your deadliest enemies need not be a nasty experience. Armed with knowledge and intelligence you can make it into something positive, even positively enjoyable—a game of skill that you can surely win. The stakes are high.

3

Are You Living Dangerously?

It may be that you are ignoring something that needs a doctor's attention.

It may be that you have habits that are potentially lethal if you don't alter them.

It may be that you are worrying too much, and harming yourself, and a reshuffling of your ideas and outlook is urgent.

It may be that a combination of circumstances in your life puts you at particular risk of one or another of the killer conditions. Knowing this will help you to counteract dangerous tendencies and sidestep serious trouble.

It is certain that there are some special points in your favor: the mitigators, that will help you to get by. It cannot help but be cheering to list these factors.

LIFE-SAVING CHECKLIST

Get out a big piece of paper and a pencil. Note the number of each statement, from the following checklist, which is true for you. For instance: *1. I am a man*. If that is what you are, put down *1*.

Are you sitting comfortably? Then check the time on your watch and go steadily through. The hodgepodge order is deliberate, to discourage you from following a trend.

1. I am a man.
2. I am a woman.
3. My work requires no special training.
4. My work requires a short training.
5. My work requires technical qualifications.
6. My work requires professional or university qualifications.
7. I travel by air fairly frequently.
8. I think that Simon and Garfunkel are a firm of solicitors.
9. I am within the ideal weight range. (See table on p. 59.)
10. I am more than 10 percent over the ideal weight range.
11. I am more than 10 percent less than the lower of the two figures on the weight chart.
12. I feel vaguely uneasy all the time.
13. I cannot run up two flights of stairs without stopping for breath. (If you haven't done this lately, put down the book and try now.)
14. I usually go out of town on weekends.
15. I sleep—or stay in bed—for more than eight hours at a stretch.
16. I have a cup of coffee/tea and a good cough for breakfast.
17. I drive peaceably. Other people think so too.
18. I don't see my children on their own for more than fifteen minutes during the week, on the average.
19. I have a dangerous job: e.g., spiderman, lion tamer, miner, bartender, cook, or journalist.
20. I can switch off and be switched on.
21. I look upon life as a challenge.
22. Basically, I'm bored.
23. My appetite is fine.

24. My appetite is good.
25. My appetite is chancy.
26. My appetite is rotten.
27. I have some varicose veins, but they don't bother me enough for me to bother about them.
28. When I am in a traffic jam I listen to the radio or try to read.
29. When I am in a traffic jam I light a cigarette and relax.
30. When I am in a traffic jam I fume.
31. I don't drive.
32. I drive more than 30,000 miles a year.
33. I get an unpleasant sensation of weight or discomfort across the chest after meals.
34. I get an unpleasant sensation of weight or discomfort across the chest after exercise.
35. I get an unpleasant sensation of weight or discomfort across the chest at any time.
36. I sleep badly; I cannot drop off.
37. I sleep badly; I wake much too early.
38. Frankly, in a bikini or bathing trunks I think I look revolting.
39. Frankly, in a bikini or bathing trunks I think I look plump.
40. Frankly, in a bikini or bathing trunks I think I look rather good.
41. Frankly, in a bikini or bathing trunks I think I look not too bad if I draw my breath in.
42. Frankly, in a bikini or bathing trunks I think I look skinny.
43. Frankly, in a bikini or bathing trunks I think I look skeletal.
44. I find my work exciting and stressful.
45. I want to get my priorities right, but they keep changing.
46. I wish I were a man/woman. (The one you aren't.)
47. I have never had jaundice.
48. I have had jaundice.
49. I sometimes notice a pain under the ribs on my right side.

50. I can flirt while walking uphill on a 1:10 gradient.
51. I guess that a push-up is a kind of bottle opener.
52. Every molehill seems like a mountain when I get to it.
53. I last saw my feet more than five years ago.
54. I've been rather lucky at times.
55. I've had pretty bad luck all my life.
56. I look forward to my retirement with dread.
57. I look forward to my retirement with longing.
58. I look forward to my retirement; I'm planning for it.
59. I am married.
60. I am single.
61. I am divorced or separated.
62. I am a widow or widower.
63. I am living in sin, long-term.
64. I see little more harm in hash than in honey for reasonably intelligent people.
65. I work fifteen hours a day, regularly
66. I know my physical and emotional limits and get help when I have reached them.
67. I have an expense account.
68. I never cry.
69. I often cry.
70. I sometimes cry (woman).
71. I rarely cry (man).
72. I love fried foods, cream, and pastries.
73. I have stomach pains in the night.
74. I feel I can't cope much longer.
75. I find sex good.
76. I find sex bad.
77. I find sex indifferent.
78. I feel I could do with a few lessons on the subject.
79. I would like to have some medical advice about it.
80. Money is one big worry.
81. I often have to entertain foreign visitors.
82. I am scared of cancer.
83. I am scared of heart disease.
84. I am scared of death.
85. When I am angry, I control it.

86. When I am angry, I work it off in physical activity.
87. When I am angry, I take it out on other people.
88. When I am angry, I swear or shout.
89. I'd rather have four lumps of sugar than one; it hasn't any taste otherwise.
90. I really enjoy making money.
91. Money isn't as important to me as other things.
92. Money is what I work for.
93. I often split my sides laughing.
94. I sometimes split my sides laughing.
95. I never split my sides laughing.
96. I enjoy the theater.
97. I enjoy music.
98. I enjoy books.
99. I enjoy watching sports.
100. I enjoy none of these.
101. Sometimes I act on a crazy impulse.
102. I'd rather have a bird than a faithful dog.
103. I have sometimes had discomfort when passing water.
104. My idea of a reviver is a brisk walk.
105. My idea of a reviver is a hot bath.
106. My idea of a reviver is a cup of coffee or tea.
107. My idea of a reviver is a few drinks.
108. My idea of a reviver is lying down for half an hour.
109. My idea of a reviver is a light meal or chocolate.
110. My idea of a reviver is phoning a friend.
111. When I walk, sometimes I get leg pains, which get better if I stop for a few moments.
112. I have had bleeding from the rectum which I assume is due to piles.
113. I don't smoke cigarettes and never have.
114. I gave them up more than a year ago.
115. I smoke a pack or less per day.
116. I smoke heavily.
117. I don't have time to sit down for breakfast.
118. I never leave my desk for lunch—I get something sent in.
119. I have stomach pains that are not helped by tablets.
120. My job is physically energetic.

121. My job requires some physical effort.
122. My job involves some moving about.
123. My job is sedentary.
124. I don't drink any alcohol.
125. I drink socially only.
126. I don't ordinarily have more than a couple of drinks a day.
127. I may have up to half a dozen drinks a day.
128. I regularly have more than this. (One drink means a single gin, whiskey or brandy, a glass of sherry or port, or a glass of beer or ale.)
129. On the whole I feel I am a good parent.

Pick your lunch from these choices:

130. Sandwich, apple pie, coffee.
131. Bread and cheese and alcoholic drink.
132. Nut salad, a glass of orange juice.
133. Lamb chop, two vegetables, cheese and crackers.
134. Shrimp cocktail, porterhouse steak and mushrooms, sautéed potatoes, cake, cheese, Turkish coffee.
135. I believe that by the year 2000 we're bound to have found some of the answers.
136. I see the end of civilized life by then.
137. I feel pretty certain of my opinions on fundamentals.
138. I feel loved by my wife/husband/children.
139. They don't care much about me.
140. I feel I am an unsuccessful parent.
141. I am subject to fainting attacks—feeling weak and sick for a few moments beforehand.
142. Sometimes my chest is wheezy.
143. My wife/husband understands me.
144. I am often nervous and irritable these days.
145. I have a dull ache on the left side of my chest, sometimes going down my arm and lasting for several hours, even days. There may be stabbing pains as well.
146. My mother is alive and well.
147. She died or is suffering from a stroke.

148. She died or is suffering from a heart attack.
149. She died or is suffering from high blood pressure.
150. She died or is suffering from diabetes.
151. She died or is suffering from something else.
152. My father is alive and well.
153. My father died at younger than fifty-five.
154. My father died or is suffering from a stroke.
155. My father died or is suffering from cancer.
156. My father died or is suffering from a heart attack.
157. My father died or is suffering from high blood pressure.
158. My father died or is suffering from diabetes.
159. My father died or is suffering from something else.
160. I have more than one relative who has died or is suffering from a stroke.
161. I have more than one relative who has died or is suffering from cancer.
162. I have more than one relative who has died or is suffering from a heart attack.
163. I have more than one relative who has died or is suffering from high blood pressure.
164. I have more than one relative who has died or is suffering from diabetes.
165. I talk about my work problems with my wife/husband.
166. I need to take aspirin or some other simple medicine every day.
167. I am on the pill.
168. I have to get up and pass water in the night, sometimes more than once.
169. I don't seem to have any energy: I'm soon tired.
170. I get pins and needles in my hands and feet.
171. I don't seem to be able to draw a satisfactory breath.
172. I have been hoarse for some time.
173. I feel full sometimes, although I have eaten nothing.
174. I have a hernia.
175. My hands and feet are often cold.
176. I prefer spicy to sweet foods.

177. I sometimes get a pain in the chest when I take a deep breath.
178. I have frequent headaches during the day.
179. I wake up with them during the night.
180. I have a cough all year round.
181. I have a cough in the winter.
182. I can discuss my problems with a friend.
183. I can never discuss my problems with a friend.
184. I look forward to the weekend with dislike.
185. I look forward to the weekend so that I can be with my family.
186. I look forward to the weekend for the change.
187. I look forward to the weekend to get some exercise.
188. I cannot stand heights, closed-in places, thunder, or something else that I know is unlikely to harm me.
189. I am sometimes conscious of my heart thumping.
190. Sometimes I have muscle spasms, e.g., my fists clench.
191. I go to church for social reasons, if ever.
192. I go to church occasionally.
193. I go to church regularly.
194. I live in a big city.
195. I live in a town.
196. I live in a rural district.
197. I know I deserve more money and appreciation than I get.

If I have an appointment a mile away and ten minutes to go:

198. I walk briskly.
199. I drive or ride.
200. I take my time.
201. I am married happily.
202. I am married tolerably.
203. I am married intolerably.
204. I'd like a change.

I play a game or do other vigorous exercise:

205. Never if I can help it.
206. Most days.
207. On weekends.
208. When I can find time.
209. My favorite breakfast is nothing or a cup of coffee or tea.
210. My favorite breakfast is an apple or other fruit and drink.
211. My favorite breakfast is cereal and milk.
212. My favorite breakfast is cereal, egg, bacon.
213. My favorite breakfast is toast or English muffins, butter, marmalade.
214. I find it difficult to concentrate.
215. I suffer from indigestion, heartburn, excessive belching or other stomach discomfort occasionally.
216. I have this kind of discomfort more often than occasionally.
217. My religion is nonexistent.
218. My religion is vague.
219. My religion is Jewish.
220. My religion is a specific Christian denomination.
221. I bring up phlegm in the mornings when I cough during the winter.
222. I have coughed up blood in the last year.
223. I have vomited blood, or altered blood (looks like coffee grounds).
224. I have passed blood in my urine, making it smoky, pink, or red.
225. I have passed blood in my stool (tarry color or red).
226. When I get into a cab I am charged double fare for extra loading.
227. I have more energy than most people: I cannot do nothing.
228. I don't have time for a real vacation.
229. I take two to three weeks' vacation each year, away from home.
230. I have six weeks' vacation or more during the year.
231. I spend some of my spare time on card games, chess, etc.

232. I spend some of my spare time on carpentry, decorating, etc.
233. I spend some of my spare time on welfare or political work.
234. I spend some of my spare time on clubs and societies.
235. I spend some of my spare time collecting stamps, antiques.
236. I spend some of my spare time on charity work.
237. I have no hobbies.
238. "A picture used in connection with a story about Solihull Hospital in last week's issue and said to be the new Accident Unit, was, in fact, the new Maternity Block." *Solihull News,* August 1970. I find that funny.
239. I don't see anything funny about that.
240. I am addicted to one of the commoner drugs: whiskey, tea, coffee, food, tobacco, etc.
241. I have irregular or postmenopausal bleeding from the vagina.
242. I know I should see my doctor, but I'm scared.
243. I am subject to muscle pains, fibrositis, or muscular rheumatism.

Now check how long you have taken to complete this list.

ANALYSIS

DANGEROUS HABITS

These numbers indicate habits or a way of life which, pursued indefinitely, could do your health irrevocable harm. If you have six or more of these numbers on your list, take it as a strong hint that your life needs reorganizing. (Make a particular study of Chapter IV.)

7, 19, 32, 38, 64, 65, 72, 89, 107, 109, 116, 118, 123, 128, 130, 134, 137, 187, 199, 205, 207, 208, 213, 226, 227, 237, 239, 240.

STITCH IN TIME

Your would be wise to consult your doctor for any *one* of these numbers. It could just mean a life saved, later— your life. Or it could mean reassurance about something that's been needling you and needn't have.

11, 26, 27, 43, 53, 73, 79, 103, 111, 112, 119, 141, 166, 168, 169, 170, 171, 173, 174, 175, 177, 179, 180, 216, 221, 222, 223, 224, 225, 241, 242. (67: Ever tried taking your *doctor* out on it?)

(DI)STRESS SIGNALS

These are signs of stress: tensions, anxieties, worries, and unpeaceful attitudes that are already affecting you adversely, and could cause you actual physical harm. They also underlie many fatal accidents. You need to learn the gentle art of relaxation and of playing it cool if you score four or more from among the following:

8, 12, 18, 22, 36, 37, 52, 55, 61, 62, 63, 68, 69, 74, 76, 78, 80, 82, 83, 84, 85, 92, 95, 100, 136, 139, 140, 141, 144, 145, 166, 171, 173, 178, 183, 184, 188, 189, 190, 203, 204, 214, 227, 228, 239, 242. (Chapter XI is especially for you.)

HAVE A HEART FOR YOUR HEART

Do you score a plus for all of these three numbers?
10, 116, 123
Then it is urgent that you make some changes. You need to work on 10, throw out 116, and take steps to counteract 123. Apart from this sinister triad any six—or more—of the following numbers suggest that you are in line for heart or artery trouble. Fortunately, there is plenty you can do to sidestep it.

10, 13, 14, 15, 24, 30, 33, 34, 35, 44, 147, 148, 149, 153, 154, 156, 157, 160, 162, 163, 170, 171, 189, 199, 207, 208, 219, 228, 240. (The next two chapters in particular are for you.)

HAVE A THOUGHT FOR:

Your Lungs

They require your special consideration if you score two or more from among these:
13, 16, 29, 171, 180, 181, 221. (Chapter VI is for you.)

Your Insulin Supplier

Diabetes is a distinct risk for everyone in the affluent society, but especially those who score two or more from among these numbers:
16, 72, 89, 130, 134, 150, 158, 164, 213, 219. (Chapter VIII is yours.)

Your Digestive System

Looks like your fueling system is feeling the strain if you score here:
19, 26, 72, 107, 134, 215, 216, 223, 225, 240. (See Chapter IX.)

Your Liver

Take particular thought for this essential organ if you score from among these:
26, 48, 49, 169, 173. (Chapter IX, again.)

Your Kidneys

Consider your kidneys if these are on your list:
103, 168, 224. (Chapter VII should be carefully read.)

LUCKY NUMBERS

You may by now have discovered that you have had habits that you should abandon, tensions that need relaxing, and areas of risk requiring tender consideration. You can do something about most of these conditions for your safety's sake, but there are other circumstances on which you can actually congratulate yourself. These are your personal lifesavers, the things that add up to a longer life. You are doing well with six or more:

2, 5, 6, 14, 17, 20, 21, 23, 28, 40, 42, 44, 45, 50, 58, 59, 66, 75, 86, 93, 94, 97, 98, 99, 101, 104, 110, 113, 114, 120, 121, 125, 129, 133, 135, 138, 146, 152, 165, 176, 182, 185, 186, 193, 195, 198, 201, 206, 229, 230, 231, 232, 233, 234, 235, 236.

For the record, if you scored any of the following numbers, here is a thought on each.

8. *Simon and Garfunkel a firm of solicitors?* If you think this sounds plausible, it seems you are not in the scene. Either you are too busy to know what is happening, or your ideas have prematurely ground to a halt. You don't have to like Simon and Garfunkel, but it's a healthy sign if you've heard of them and haven't stepped irrevocably into the outlook of middle age.

18. *I don't see my kids on their own for more than fifteen minutes.* Whatever else you're doing, you are missing out on living. Seems your priorities have slipped.

56. *I look forward to my retirement with dread.* If you don't want it to kill you outright, you had better start developing some interests in your work and your leisure that will carry you on.

67. *I have an expense account.* Dangerous privilege— can't you trade it in for a bicycle? Or bribe a particular restaurant to feed you nothing but rabbit food, no matter what your guests have, and regardless of what you order.

82, 83, 84. *I am scared of cancer, heart disease, death.* Fine, that's good motivation to do something positive. Read on to find out what.

P.S. *The time factor:* If you took around ten minutes to make your list, and it was legible, that is average. If you took six minutes or less, then your notion of taking it easy needs decelerating, or you'll spend your life tensed up like a sprinter. Fifteen minutes or more might indicate that you are tired, depressed, or taking your health a little too seriously.

*Table of Desirable Weights**
Age 25 and Over

Weight in pounds (in indoor clothing)
Men

Height (in shoes)†	Small frame	Medium frame	Large frame
5 ft. 2 in.	112-120	118-129	126-141
5 ft. 3 in.	115-123	121-133	129-144
5 ft. 4 in.	118-126	124-136	132-148
5 ft. 5 in.	121-129	127-139	135-152
5 ft. 6 in.	124-133	130-143	138-150
5 ft. 7 in.	128-137	134-147	142-161
5 ft. 8 in.	132-141	138-153	147-166
5 ft. 9 in.	136-145	142-156	151-170
5 ft. 10 in.	140-150	146-160	155-174
5 ft. 11 in.	144-154	150-165	159-179
6 ft. 0 in.	148-158	154-170	164-184
6 ft. 1 in.	152-162	158-175	168-189
6 ft. 2 in.	156-167	162-180	173-194
6 ft. 3 in.	160-171	167-185	178-199
6 ft. 4 in.	164-175	172-190	182-204

Women

	Small frame	Medium frame	Large frame
4 ft. 10 in.	92-98	96-107	104-119
4 ft. 11 in.	94-101	98-110	106-122
5 ft. 0 in.	96-104	101-113	109-125
5 ft. 1 in.	99-107	104-116	112-128
5 ft. 2 in.	102-110	107-119	115-131
5 ft. 3 in.	105-113	110-122	118-134
5 ft. 4 in.	108-116	113-126	121-138
5 ft. 5 in.	111-119	116-130	125-142
5 ft. 6 in.	114-123	120-135	129-146
5 ft. 7 in.	118-127	124-139	133-150
5 ft. 8 in.	122-131	128-143	137-154
5 ft. 9 in.	126-135	132-147	141-158
5 ft. 10 in.	130-140	136-151	145-163
5 ft. 11 in.	134-144	140-155	149-168
6 ft. 0 in.	138-148	144-159	153-174

* Those associated with longest life. Note that these weights are less than the Average Weights. Notice too that desirable adult weight remains the same throughout adulthood from age 25, whereas average weights rise to a maximum at ages 50–59.

† 1-inch heels for men and 2-inch heels for women.

Table of Average Weights

Weight in pounds (in indoor clothing)

Men

Height (in shoes)*	Ages 20-24	Ages 25-29	Ages 30-39	Ages 40-49	Ages 50-59	Ages 60-69
5 ft. 2 in.	128	134	137	140	142	139
5 ft. 3 in.	132	138	141	144	145	142
5 ft. 4 in.	136	141	145	148	149	146
5 ft. 5 in.	139	144	149	152	153	150
5 ft. 6 in.	142	148	153	156	157	154
5 ft. 7 in.	145	151	157	161	162	159
5 ft. 8 in.	149	155	161	165	166	163
5 ft. 9 in.	153	159	165	169	170	168
5 ft. 10 in.	157	163	170	174	175	173
5 ft. 11 in.	161	167	174	178	180	178
6 ft. 0 in.	166	172	179	183	185	183
6 ft. 1 in.	170	177	183	187	189	188
6 ft. 2 in.	174	183	188	192	194	193
6 ft. 3 in.	178	186	193	197	199	198
6 ft. 4 in.	181	190	199	203	205	204

Women

	Ages 20-24	Ages 25-29	Ages 30-39	Ages 40-49	Ages 50-59	Ages 60-69
4 ft. 10 in.	102	107	115	122	125	127
4 ft. 11 in.	105	110	117	124	127	129
5 ft. 0 in.	108	113	120	127	130	131
5 ft. 1 in.	112	116	123	130	133	134
5 ft. 2 in.	115	119	126	133	136	137
5 ft. 3 in.	118	122	129	136	140	141
5 ft. 4 in.	121	125	132	140	144	145
5 ft. 5 in.	125	129	135	143	148	149
5 ft. 6 in.	129	133	139	147	152	153
5 ft. 7 in.	132	136	142	151	156	157
5 ft. 8 in.	136	140	146	158	160	161
5 ft. 9 in.	140	144	150	159	164	165
5 ft. 10 in.	144	148	154	164	169	†
5 ft. 11 in.	149	153	159	169	174	†
6 ft. 0 in.	154	158	164	174	180	†

* 1-inch heels for men and 2-inch heels for women.
† Average weights not determined because of insufficient data.

4

Loading the Dice
in Your Favor

They taught you a lot of stuff in school about literature
and mathematics, science and the arts: they may even
have touched on the birds and the bees. But it's a safe bet
that they didn't include any lessons in living. Yet the basic
rudiments of survival comprise a complex subject in today's man-made environment, and need intelligent study.
It is useful to know how to function effectively without
damaging your personal machinery.

When earning a living meant hunting or farming, there
was no difficulty over holding the diet at a safe level or
taking adequate exercise. Stress was something straightforward, like a wild animal coming for you, and instinct
told you all you needed to know. Now the hunter has only
to dip his hand into the deep freeze, and earning one's
daily bread means, for many of us, sitting at a desk. Even
a working housewife has little use for muscle power, with
electricity at her elbow. You are more likely to move
around on wheels than to walk, and you merely throw a
switch for entertainment. Noise is your constant and nerve-
jangling companion, and competition in the business arena
is fiercer than living by the sword ever was.

You are, in today's different world, using bodily equipment designed some five hundred thousand years ago, and not modified since. It's like taking a one-cylinder Oldsmobile of 1902 vintage for a spin on a roaring modern motorway. It stands to reason that you must apply knowledge and skill to get the best out of the machine.

Your body is 30 percent muscle, 15 percent bone and 2 percent brain. That gives you the relative importance of these components in the original model. The only recent change is that it has become fashionable to replace some of the muscle by fat—and then add some more. Living is made up of work and relaxation, eating and exercise, sleeping and sex: the optimum proportions of each spell happiness and health.

Take work: it's what enables most of us to live at all. Even a junkie will do enough for his needs. Work helps your health by financing your food and shelter. It may also involve healthful physical exertion: the harder the more beneficial. Among longshoremen in New England and London Transport employees in old England, those with the more energetic jobs have the better record for reaching retirement age. It may bore you, but it won't kill you to work with your muscles. It won't keep you awake at night, worrying, either.

Brain work, on the other hand, has the advantage of possibly not feeling like work at all. The ideal job, they say, is something you'd pay to be allowed to do—if you could afford it. The danger is that you may get hooked, and work addiction is as deadly as heroin addiction, particularly if it is stressful. It is noteworthy—if you are at a crossroads in your career—that scientists stand 20 percent less chance of dying young than other professional people, and college professors and administrators some 10 to 15 percent less. Correspondents and journalists run more than twice the average risk of early death, while writers as a group have a 30 percent poorer chance than others to live. Doctors rate much the same as journalists. In Britain, Members of Parliament have a lower than average likelihood of dying too soon, except from a coronary, but presidential candidates in the United States, successful or unsuccessful, have shorter lives than most, even putting assassination aside.

The outlook for businessmen varies: for instance, those who are university graduates tend to be tougher, as far as survival goes, than those who are "self-made." But they are all likely to be neck-deep in a psychologically tense, sedentary life, with its added dangers of "working lunches," rather than living the safer, standoff life of the academic or administrative man or woman. *The deadly delusion of indispensability is particularly prevalent in the business world.*

Or the money trap: "I know I'm killing myself with overwork, but I'm making so much I can afford it. . . ."

Outside interests and activities act as an antidote to overwork and make for a healthy balance. Omar Sharif, who leads a life of lurid adventure on film, is a bridge player of international repute off the set. Churchill painted watercolors and built a brick wall when he wasn't running a war. If you are inside, sitting down all day at work, you ought to get outdoors and into something physical to counteract the effects of inactivity. The same principle holds for your vacation.

If your work creates tensions, it is all the more urgent that you develop a good unwinding technique—usually through other interests. But if you are already so sold on your job that you can't conceive of anything that isn't connected with it worth doing, fool yourself this way. Choose one aspect of your work, preferably outside the mainstream, approach it more leisurely, with the pleasure principle in mind, and count that as your hobby. If vacations frustrate and bore you, plan them around something that has to do with your subject—even if it's only a pilgrimage to the burial place of the last colleague of yours to buy a coronary. Any letup from an accelerating work treadmill is life-saving, and will keep you at it longer in the end.

A good vacation can do a lot to balance out six months of exhausting work, if you use some wit in making your arrangements. If you are normally in a tearing hurry, don't try to do Europe in six days. Meander. If you live well in the ordinary way, and have a fat expense account, go for the simple life in the wilds. If you can afford to have help in your home, don't take an effort-free cruise. If you live in the polluted atmosphere of a big city 90 percent of your breathing time, go where there's clean air to wash out your lungs.

But: if you have physically loafed all year, you are asking for disaster if you go in for a few weeks' strenuous exercise without giving your heart and lungs warning of the extra demands to be made upon them. Some of my best friends, and maybe yours, have killed themselves by trying to pack into one month the exercise for twelve, or even that for a week into a weekend. You need a base of fitness in order for an active vacation to build up your health. Another fatal fallacy of vacations is "getting your money's worth"—particularly common among the male sex. It usually means eating more than you want because "it's included." But it is poor value to harm your health, just because you've paid for the privilege.

You should have more sense than that. It's a matter of statistical fact that outstanding men, for instance those in the American *Who's Who,* are not in the habit of dying young. Their mortality rates at forty-five to forty-nine, fifty to fifty-four, and fifty-five to fifty-nine years of age are only about half those of other white men of the same age in the United States. It could be that they are all blessed with a remarkable constitution from the cradle, but it may also be that they use some of their time and initiative on preventive maintenance of their most valuable assets for success: themselves. Even Billy Graham, to be seen jogging around Hyde Park whenever he visits London, doesn't leave it all to luck and the Lord.

DIET

Eating and exercise are among the most important facets of living for your bodily well-being. Like work and play, they are two sides of the same coin—opposites in some ways, yet they go together.

Eating and drinking comprise the intake of nutrients that is essential for all body processes: for keeping you warm by slow internal combustion; for powering your muscle force, including your heart and breathing muscles; for repair and regeneration of worn and damaged tissues; for the normal processing in the digestive factories; and, in minute quantities only, for your brain's activities. This latter point is one of the pitfalls of the seventies. Modern occupations employ brains and machinery rather than muscle energy, and requirements for food must be reassessed downward continually, as this trend develops.

In order to discuss eating you must first understand the jargon:

Calorie (strictly, *kilocalorie*): This is a measure of the nourishing power of food, related to the amount of heat it could produce if burned. A slice of bread, an egg, or a one-inch cube of Cheddar cheese provides you with about one hundred calories—to use for body processes or to be stored as fat.

Proteins, fats, and carbohydrates are the basic constituents of food.

Proteins: Found mainly in meat, fish, poultry, cheese, eggs, peas, and beans. They are expensive, but in the affluent West, the 6 percent proportion of protein in the diet that is necessary for health is usually doubled. Excess protein can be converted into body fat, but less readily than the other two types of food.

Fats: Oily and greasy foods. They are of two types: *saturated,* usually from animal sources and solid at room temperature; and *polyunsaturated,* usually from vegetable oils, like sassafras. The latter help to reduce the amount in the blood of the animal-fat derivative *cholesterol,* which appears to be connected with atherosclerosis.

Carbohydrates: Foods derived from plants are basically carbohydrate. It is an excess of carbohydrates that most commonly leads to life-shortening obesity, and they are in particular to be found in the refined products of Western industrialism: sugar, breakfast cereals, white bread and flour.

Calorie ratings: i.e., nourishing or fattening power:

Each gram of protein you eat provides 4 calories.
Each gram of carbohydrate you eat provides 4 calories.
Each gram of fat you eat provides 9 calories.
Each gram of alcohol you drink provides 7 calories.

The official recommendations on the amount of food that is desirable for health today are as follows:

United States
   Men: 2800 calories daily, tapering to 2400 by age 55.
   Women: 2000 calories daily, tapering to 1700 by age 55.
Britain
   Men: 3000 calories daily, tapering to 2500 by age 55.
   Women: 2200 calories daily, tapering to 2050 by age 55.

The difference between the two countries is because of the excess of cars, elevators, mechanization, and central heating in the United States.

An intake of food that would have been barely adequate fifty years ago would leave today's average man with a dangerous surplus. If you take aboard more nourishment than your body needs for its day-to-day energy output, you run the risk of storing the rest as fat. This doesn't invariably happen, as the body has a mechanism called *thermogenesis* for burning away the surplus. It is more effective in some individuals than in others, and generally in the adolescent more than the adult, the male more than the female. It is this mechanism that allows some people to eat twice as much as others and yet remain irritatingly lean. However, this doesn't help your problem if you are what they call a *good* converter—not an evangelist, but one who has the power to convert every spare morsel of food into fat.

Fat is first deposited in and around the abdomen, then as a layer over the whole body, finally infiltrating every tissue and organ, including the walls of the essential pipe-lines, the arteries.

Obesity, defined as a 10 percent or more increase over the desirable weight for your height, sex, and age, is the commonest disease in our culture and as far-reaching in its effects on your body as a cancer. For every 10 percent of weight over the desired weight you clip 13 percent off your life expectancy. For the average man, twenty-five pounds too many at age fifty means that, instead of looking forward to another twenty years, he should plan on fifteen. If, at forty, you are fifty pounds fatter than you should be, you needn't plan for your retirement at all: the chances are that you'll never make it. Check your situation by looking at the chart on p. 68.

Fat deposits are the visible signs of an invisible killer. The most damaging effects of obesity are likely to be on your heart and arteries, though atherosclerosis, coronary disease, thrombosis and embolism, and high blood pressure. Your heart has to labor harder, night and day, to pump through the extra adipose tissue: the pressure must go up to achieve this, and this, in turn, reacts on the heart itself. The risk of stroke, from an artery giving way under the strain, is greater. Raised blood pressure also puts your kidneys at risk: their delicate mechanism works best at a normal pressure range.

Your chest will be at a disadvantage in any infection, acute or chronic, if its movements are hampered by a heavy wrapping of fat. There's a much greater likelihood of your developing diabetes if you are fat—it seems that you can exhaust your body's powers of coping with too much sugar in the blood. Cirrhosis of the liver, that outsider that's coming up on the rail to fifth place in the United States mortality stakes, is more prevalent in the obese. So are diseases of the gall bladder, including gallstones; complications in pregnancy and childbirth; and postoperative disasters; and you are *automatically* classed as a bad anesthetic risk if you are fat.

Among obesity-linked disorders that don't kill directly are rheumatoid and osteoarthritis, slipped disk, varicose veins, and diaphragmatic hernia; infertility is commoner in the obese of either sex; if you are heavy and ungainly, you cannot leap out of the way of an oncoming truck too nimbly, and if you have a fall it will be heavier. Excess fat in your bloodstream means reduced efficiency—not only physically but mentally. The unattractive, sleepy Fat Boy of *The Pickwick Papers* was an extreme example of this. Fat people tend to sleep longer, and this in itself is not healthy, as we shall see.

Obesity is a dangerous disease, but fortunately it is slow-acting, and eminently capable of reversal, without surgery, expense, special drugs, or apparatus. If you are a woman the effects of obesity are as harmful to you as they are to a man in the long run, but the run is longer. Up until menopause a woman can carry off a certain "curvaceousness" without incurring the dangers that beset a man, but even so, she is safer being slim.

WHAT DO THE FATTIES DIE FROM?

	Cause of Death	Percentage of risk increase because of obesity
Men	Heart disease, including coronary attack and angina	42
	Stroke	59
	Kidney disease	90
	Diabetes	283
	Pneumonia	2
	Cirrhosis of the liver	49
	Hernia and obstruction	54
	Gallstones	106
	Car accidents	31
Women	Heart disease, including coronary attack and angina	75
	Stroke	62
	Kidney disease	112
	Cancer of the womb	21
	Diabetes	272
	Pneumonia	29
	Cirrhosis of the liver	47
	Hernia and obstruction	41
	Gallstones	184
	Childbirth	61
	Car accidents	20

As recently as the 1930's, insurance companies gave preferential treatment to the slightly overweight! The one bright spot in the survival of the fattest is their consistently low suicide rates: about 25 percent lower than the average for either sex.

The central error leading to obesity is in the input/output accounting. Various factors can get it off balance: the wide variety of attractive, concentrated foods that take neither time nor trouble to prepare and are within the means of all who are affluent; the fact that brain men are better paid than muscle men, who are becoming obsolete with mechanization; different habits. Wesley walked fifteen miles every Sunday, through the smiling Cornish countryside, just to hear a second sermon: we ride to our work in undesirable stressful conditions when it may be no more than two miles. Paradoxically, in our society it is looked upon as lazy to walk when you might clip a few minutes' traveling time by riding.

Professional men—on the whole—are fatter than manual workers, but their wives, with greater combined fashion-and-fitness sense, are slimmer than less well-to-do women.

Appestatics: What should naturally control the amount you eat, and gear it to your requirements, is your appetite, regulated from the brain by the *appestat*. If you burn more fuel because of muscle work or to keep warm, your appestat will put your appetite up a notch. But if your physical activity is minimal and your surroundings centrally heated, your appestat may not be able to register low enough. It's difficult, similarly, to make your car run smoothly at two miles an hour. Unless your muscles are used to a certain extent, your appestat cannot work efficiently.

This can apply to anyone, but it applies more strongly in the mesomorphic types—those built for physical energy and go-getting, who have often been athletic in their college days. These are the natural candidates for the Coronary Club, if they don't take care of their appestats, their diets, and their exercising. Others, who easily became plump, even in childhood, but were never very wonderful at sports, the charming, sociable endomorphs, are slightly less liable to coronary attacks. Fat women tend to be of this type. The people least likely to be troubled by overweight, the kind who eat huge platefuls of meat, yet who always look slight, are the angular ectomorphs.

Another factor that acts unfairly is thermogenesis, the burning off of surplus nutriment. But for almost everyone, increasing age—once past twenty-five—reduces the efficiency of thermogenesis and at the same time brings more responsible, more sedentary work.

If the scales read DANGER: It is no matter for fatalism or despair if you find that you have become fat or are showing early warnings. This is something you can put right yourself. Whatever the predisposing causes, the basic fact remains that you are getting more food than your body can use. You can adjust this. You are unlikely to quit your job to take up lumberjacking or mining coal, and the amount of exercise you can fit into your spare time wouldn't even scratch the surface of the problem. It would take a hundred holes of golf, twenty sets of tennis, or a fifty-mile hike to burn up a single pound of body fat. Exercise has other benefits to health and a modicum is necessary to get your appestat operating, but the main thrust of your attack on obesity must be through diet.

Dieting is not synonymous with near-starvation. Dieting means eating, eating intelligently. At a conference I attended recently I happened to sit next to a lady who had lost 112 pounds in the last eight months, by diet alone. Yet she told me, "I eat more now than I ever did when I was fat." She was a member of Weight Watchers International, the fatties' organization that straddles the Atlantic and helps the overweight to help themselves, with more lasting success than any other system to date. WW programs include neither drugs nor exercises, but planned eating—plus encouragement, comradeship, and rewards. There's likely to be a WW group near you, or you may get your doctor to plan a program for you, or you may prefer to "do it yourself." Whichever way you play it, you'll be doing the hard part yourself anyway.

OUR PLAN, FOR YOU

1. *Make a frank assessment of the situation.* Look at yourself in a full-length mirror; do you look flabby? A muscular person may weigh as much as a fat one and be perfectly fit. Pick up a fold of skin over your lower ribs: if it is more than a quarter-inch thick then you are too plump. The same test can be done with more sophistication by skin-fold calipers or ultrasonic probe. Next: weigh yourself and check with the chart of desirable weights, p. 59.

2. *Decide on your target weight.*

3. *At this point,* if you have twenty pounds or more to shed, or have doubts about your fitness, consult your doctor on the advisability of dieting. You will probably receive his blessing. If so:

4. *Get going.* Today, not tomorrow or after Christmas. Make a note of your present weight, and repeat weekly, wearing the same clothing. More frequent weigh-ins will give you some interesting sidelights on daily variations due to bowel movements, etc., but may alternately cheer and depress you.

5. *Choose your weapons.* Either:

   a. Eat as you always have, but cut the portions in half. If you are capable of dividing by two, you will certainly get slimmer. *Or:*

   b. Pick your day's diet from one of the diets below. Each one allows a little over 1000 calories, about half what you need for the day's fueling: the rest must come off you.

   c. Play a game of instead-of, according to the rules below.

SAMPLE DIETS

No added sugar. *No* alcohol.

A. BREAKFAST
Half grapefruit; 2 slices grilled lean bacon; 1 slice plain
bread; coffee or tea with milk.

LUNCH
4 ounces cottage cheese; salad of cucumber and lettuce; 1 Ry-Krisp; apple; coffee.

DINNER
Small glass tomato juice; grilled lean lamb chop; green
beans and carrots; orange segments and plain yogurt; coffee.

B. BREAKFAST
Scrambled egg; broiled tomato; 1 slice toast; tea or
coffee with milk.

LUNCH
3 fish sticks, oven-heated; peas; glass of skim milk.

DINNER
Clear soup; stewed beef, Brussels sprouts; stewed
fruit (no sugar) and semisweet wafer; coffee.

C. BREAKFAST
1 ounce cheese, melted on toast; orange, whole; tea or
coffee with milk.

LUNCH
Cold, lean meats; watercress and tomato; pear; 1
cracker; coffee.

DINNER
Grilled liver; spinach; rye biscuit; fresh fruit salad;
coffee.

D. BREAKFAST
Stewed prunes and wheat germ; thinly margarined slice of toast; coffee or tea with milk.

LUNCH
Egg; cauliflower; 1-inch cube of cheese and apple; coffee.

DINNER
Slice of melon; roast beef or lamb; Brussels sprouts; tangerine; coffee.

E. BREAKFAST
Poached haddock; slice of thinly margarined bread; ½ orange; tea or coffee with milk.

LUNCH
Plain omelette; watercress; other half of orange; semi-sweet wafer; coffee.

DINNER
Grilled steak; mushrooms; cooked tomatoes; fresh fruit in season; coffee.

F. BREAKFAST
Grated raw apple with cottage cheese; 1 piece rye or wheat melba toast; coffee.

LUNCH
Sardines on dry toast; salad; apple; coffee.

DINNER
Chicken casserole with mixed vegetables (no potatoes); banana; coffee.

G. BREAKFAST
Half grapefruit; boiled egg; slice of plain bread; coffee.

LUNCH
4 ounces salmon; lettuce and cucumber; plums or
grapes; plain cracker; coffee.

DINNER
Braised ham and celery, or endive; plain yogurt; coffee.

PLAYING INSTEAD-OF

Instead of	Take
Sugar	Artificial sweetener
Soda pop or Coke	Low-calorie soft drink
Cream cheese	Cottage cheese
Jam, jelly, honey	Cheese or meat spreads
Sweet pickles	Pickled cabbage, dill pickles, cucumbers
Thick sauces	Worcestershire sauce, mustard
Breakfast cereals	Unsugared stewed fruit
Puddings and pies	Fresh fruit
Sausages	Fish sticks, no batter
Peas	Spinach
Bananas	Oranges
Avocado	Pears
Ice cream	Low-fat, unsweetened yogurt
Crackers	Celery
Butter	Margarine
Packaged Jell-O	Unsweetened gelatin flavored with fruit juice
Fried foods	Grilled, boiled, baked, steamed foods
Bacon, pork, ham	Veal, beef, lamb

You can work out your own variations on the theme,
given the clues:

Harmless foods: Clear soups, meat extracts, lean meat,
fish, eggs, chicken (no skin), turkey, rabbit, hare, green-
leaf vegetables, tomatoes, tomato juice, cheese (not cream

cheese), nuts, fresh fruit (not bananas), salads, chicory, celery, asparagus, lettuce, tea, coffee, low-calorie carbonated drinks, gelatin, spices.

O.K. once or twice a week: Beef, liver, salmon, all-beef frankfurters.

Have as little as possible of these: Bread and everything made with flour, cereals, including breakfast cereals and puddings, starchy vegetables, sugar, and foods containing sugar, sweets, puddings, pastries, cakes and sauces, alcohol, "diabetic" jams, malted-milk drinks, soda pop, more than one cup of milk daily.

Note: If you are trying to maintain a low blood cholesterol level, that changes the diet picture slightly. See below.

6. *Take each day as it comes, and make the best of it.*

7. *Get the cooperation of your wife/husband.* The dangerous period for most men begins when the wedding is over. The more loving the wife, the more dangerous. But encouragement, exhortation, and mild reproof when necessary do help strengthen one's resolve.

8. *Never miss a meal.* There's a beneficial—to you— thermic effect from having a meal. It speeds up your metabolism, the rate at which your body's chemical processes proceed, and by which it burns up food or fat. It used to be thought that only proteins had this thermic effect: now it is known that all foods act the same way.

9. *Get the bonus effect of exercise after a meal.* The thermic effect of a meal is doubled by muscular activity immediately following, so more surplus is burned off. A dinner dance makes good sense physiologically, and so does a walk to the station after breakfast. It's a pity that business lunches don't wind up with a cha-cha.

10. *Avoid the bad habit of night eating.* Don't take your main meal very late in the evening, after a show, for instance, or grab a calorific snack before bed—especially if there is no one else in the kitchen. If you have your night's rest with a loaded stomach you absorb every scrap of nourishment—to convert into fat, rather than muscle energy and warmth, which you don't need in bed.

11. *Live cool.* Have minimal bed covering, low-set thermostats, and light clothes. This will make your body provide some of its own central heating, and it will burn its internal fuel faster.

12. *Alcohol is out during the reducing period.* Not only does it contribute substantially to caloric intake (nearly twice as fattening as sugar, gram for gram) but it is difficult to take a drink before dinner and retain your will power intact during the meal. It's asking for failure.

Later, when your weight is about right, and all you need do is keep it steady, you may be able to enjoy the occasional social drink, instead of something else. Figure your calculations from the following data:

An ordinary two-ounce glass of sherry, a liqueur glass of Benedictine or the like, a single whiskey, rum, gin, or vodka, each rates at about sixty to seventy calories, much the same as a poached egg or a serving of peas.

A glass of champagne is equivalent, in fattening power, to a couple of oranges or a slice of bread and butter.

Half a pint of beer counts the same as a glass of champagne, but pale ale is more nourishing, and stout, or strong ale, doubly so.

Cider is more fattening than ale, and hard cider the worst alcoholic drink of all—for the dieter.

Dry varieties of drink, including sherries and ciders, are less calorific than sweet.

Red Beaujolais and Chianti are wiser table wines for you than the sweet and the white; but if it must be white, choose a dry one.

OTHER METHODS OF WEIGHT REDUCTION (TO EXAMINE AND DISCARD)

1. *Turkish and sauna baths,* massage, sauna pants, colonic washouts—all achieve a temporary loss of fluid and therefore of weight, which is soon replaced. They

don't rid you of any of your harmful fat. Useless, and occasionally dangerous in themselves.

2. *Slimming drugs:* Amphetamines curb your appetite and pep you up, but they can cause headaches, high blood pressure, and severe mental disturbances. They are addictive and best left alone. Thyroxine doesn't work unless you are thyroid-deficient, or take it in such high dosage that it might damage your heart. Fenfluramine is said to mobilize your body fat, but it slows you down and may clash with other drugs. Unless your doctor absolutely approves, don't bother with these forlorn hopes.

3. *Fillers:* Methyl cellulose tablets, wafers, soups, etc., swell up in your stomach but they don't leave you feeling satisfied, so they are not effective in reducing appetite.

4. *Sedatives and tranquilizers:* These have no place in a slimming regimen per se, but if you are overeating because of anxieties, suppressed aggression, or depression, they may help. It's more to the point to come to terms with what's eating you.

5. *Diuretics:* Drugs that stimulate you into passing water reduce your weight temporarily if it is due to excess fluid in the tissues. No effect on excess fat.

6. *Plastic surgery:* Can produce overnight temporary improvement, but except occasionally, as in the case of enormous (female) breasts, the final appearance may well be worse than the original. New fat tends to be deposited in irregular lumps, and from the health angle there is immediate danger from the release of fat globules into the bloodstream. The other operation tried at one time for obesity was the "short circuiting" of part of the intestine; dangerous.

7. *Crash diets and complete starvation:* These can be dangerous if used for long, and the latter has led to several deaths. Besides, in most cases the weight lost by such dramatic means is soon regained. A regular one-day-a-week fast, however, can be useful for holding the weight steady while eating normally the rest of the time.

8. *Gimmicky diets,* like oranges and peanuts, milk and bananas, and commercially prepared cans of carefully balanced nutrients of a certain caloric value may work

temporarily, but are impracticable for a lifetime of healthy weight.

9. *Injections to redistribute your fat:* don't.

10. *Cutting down on salt and water* makes little difference to the fat on your body, though it might relieve you of excess fluid.

11. *Cutting out mealtime drinking* has no effect except possibly to limit the amount of dry, salty, or spicy food you can enjoy at a meal.

None of these ploys acts effectively. The only way to achieve and keep a healthy weight is to learn the rules of wise eating, and retrain your tastes to conform to them; this takes about four months. But it is more efficient than removing your surplus weight rapidly, and then putting it on again even faster—the roller-coaster system that gets you nowhere.

SUMMATION

EAT LOTS OF FRUIT AND VEGETABLES.

BE RUTHLESS IN REFUSING WHAT'S DEATH TO YOU.

NEVER EAT AT NIGHT.

NEVER MISS A MEAL.

BE ACTIVE AFTER EATING.

En route to your goal: in the first week or two you may be gratified by the loss of several pounds with comparatively little effort. This is as likely due to a change in your water balance as well as to actual loss of fat, so don't be dismayed when the same diet doesn't seem to produce such good results a week later. If you achieve a steady loss of two or three pounds a week you are doing excellently. Keep at it. Unfortunately, fat, as we've seen, is the most concentrated form of body fuel, so it takes time to rid yourself of surplus stores.

When you've arrived at your "target" weight, continue

with your weekly weighings, just to make sure that your books are balanced and that input is not overtaking output. You know what to do at the first hint; and it's easier to check a tendency than to peel off a large excess.

WHAT ABOUT CHOLESTEROL?

Cholesterol is a fat derivative which is synthesized in the body and also obtained direct from certain foods. Cholesterol in the right quantity is, like blood pressure, essential to life. But a higher than normal amount in the blood has a sinister association with atherosclerosis, the commonest killer of the day. You may choose to go warily with foods containing a substantial amount of this material; this is a separate matter from slimming. Although fat people almost all have unhealthily high blood cholesterol, others, who are distinctly lean, may yet have dangerously high cholesterol levels as well.

The common high-cholesterol foods include: bacon, ham, butter, drippings, egg yolk, cheese, Spam, sausages, pork, brains, oysters, and animal fats in general.

Polyunsaturated vegetable (not nut) oils, such as corn oil, and fish oils are available in soft margarines and for cooking. Eating these helps to reduce the amount of cholesterol in the blood more than merely cutting down the cholesterol intake. It is wise for most men to choose to take some polyunsaturated fat in their meals. Such fats are not "slimming," but by soothing the stomach even more than some animal fats, they may make you feel comfortable for a longer time after eating, and so help you to eat less altogether.

Brown or whole-meal bread contains polyunsaturated wheat-germ oil, and also part of the vitamin B complex which the body needs to enable it to utilize vegetable oils. It is a better choice than the modern, emasculated white bread from which both of these substances have been eliminated.

FOOD YOU MUST HAVE

Don't fall into the error of thinking that all food is poison, and eating a sin. You must eat, if moderately, to live. Man is omnivorous and needs, above all, variety; it is the lack of this commodity that makes some diets dangerous. You need to take daily some protein, some fat, and some carbohydrate. You need foods that contain the principal vitamins and minerals. Vitamins A and D are contained in margarine, carrots, and fish oil, and you can synthesize D in your own skin with the help of sunshine. Vitamin C is freely available in fresh fruits and salads; vitamins B and E are present in wheat germ, yeast, and liver. All of these vitamins are better utilized by the body when they come from food rather than from special concentrates.

EXERCISE

Exercise is a useful adjunct to your weight-control program, mainly by raising your energy output sufficiently for your appestat—appetite control—to operate. Take a look at the slimming value of various activities:

Calories Burned Per Hour

Just existing	67 (men)
	56 (women)
Plus:	
Sitting, viewing or listening	15
Standing	35
Typing	40
Office work	20–220
Heavy work, men	375–550
Hard housework	150–300
Light housework	80–120
Gardening	200–400
Ping-pong	100–200
Football	350

Tennis	250–350
Walking slowly	120
Walking at 5 mph up 1:10 hill	850
Making a bed	350
Swimming	400
Washing dishes	40
Dancing	250–350
Coal mining	550

However, whether you are fat or lean, exercise, in its own right, is vitally important to your health. Some doctors consider it the most important single factor for survival. It makes you stronger and better-looking, which boosts your morale. It makes you more resistant to psychological strains. It peps up your mental alertness through better circulation and improves your resistance to physical stress. It helps you to keep warm in winter and to sleep soundly in any season. It helps to prevent or cure backache. In particular, it benefits your heart, arteries, and lungs—the most precious parts of your machinery for living.

Exercising your body muscles automatically puts your heart and lungs through a training course so that they may provide the greater circulatory output and oxygen intake required.

Exercise needs to be taken daily to be safe and effective. Weekend splurges of activity, such as mowing lawns and other forms of sport, are too frequently followed by an obituary in Monday's papers. But you *can* make yourself physically fit, and stay that way, partly by taking every opportunity for exercise during your normal day.

If you feel like getting up from your chair and pacing up and down, do it.

If you can't sleep, react by taking a stroll.

Walk when you might ride; walk tall, brisk, springily. Try breathing in for six paces, out for six: work up to ten.

Climb stairs when you might use an elevator. Don't use the handrail, and take them two, three, and four at a time: fine for your heart, lungs, and hip joints.

Indoors, walk with your heels hardly touching the ground, and at every opportunity try a few heel raises.

Sit tall, with your back straight, as a habit: it'll impress your boss or business adversary, too.

Housework: don't let anyone deprive you of the beneficial activity. Do it at a swinging tempo, to the radio.

Sit down and stand up without leaning on your desk or chair—the lower the chair the better.

Do desk push-ups: hands flat on the desk, elbows bent, try to lift yourself up by pressing down.

Towel yourself after a shower so that your muscles are glowing inside as well as your skin outside.

When you are doing something mechanical, like driving a car, routine work, or telephoning your husband or wife, tense your abdominal muscles in six-second bursts: it actually improves your mental efficiency by increasing the blood supply to the brain. Practice pressing your knees together. Contract one buttock, then the other. Or press down with your hands and push your knees up against them, feet on tiptoe under the desk.

Stretch like a cat, with or without a yawn.

All this is very fine, but you also need a definite daily dose of heart-muscle-lung tonic.

Daily is the key word: or nearly every day. After a recent garbage men's strike in London, men who had never found it any effort to lift heavy garbage cans before were sweating and breathless on the job, after three weeks' idleness. An hour's daily walking at a brisk pace is fine health insurance, and unlikely to do you any harm, whatever your condition or age. Or you can join the dawn-and-dusk brigade of joggers who are to be found in every big city. The usual routine is to walk a block and jog a block alternately for a fifteen-minute stint, night and morning.

Games and sports provide social benefits as well as just exercise, and they may be more interesting. But they are not always easy for a city dweller to fit in, and such games as squash are too violent for safety if you play them past forty, unless you train yourself slowly. Of course, social drinking afterward may undo much of the good the game has done, or a fiercely competitive spirit may produce as much tension as big business. A further disadvantage of most sports is that they don't condition the whole body, although swimming comes near to it.

The most compact method of fighting city dweller's flab is by a system of formal exercises tailored to fit into fifteen minutes of your day. Essentials are to employ a wide range of movements so as to use as many muscles and joints as possible, and on an increasing scale. This is the basis of any training scheme, including your training for survival, and when you have achieved a satisfactory level of physical fitness you must continue to exercise to maintain it.

If you decide on a specialized, streamlined course, the Royal Canadian Air Force eleven-minute-a-day 5BX program for men, and the twelve-minute XBX program for women, are among the most widely used. They require no apparatus, and no more space than you need to lie down. Warming up is an integral part of the system; and done according to instructions, these exercises involve no danger of exhaustion or overstrain. However, 5BX can kill—and it has—when used wrongly. The big temptation is to start halfway through, or skip to the end, to astronaut standard, which is as much cheating as peeking at the last page of a novel first—and much more risky.

DO-IT-YOURSELF METHOD

Take a handful of the following exercises and do them, in order, while you listen to a favorite radio program that runs about fifteen minutes. Don't do anything that feels a strain: this means that as a beginner you will be able to do more of the first three than of the next two exercises; with the last two it's a matter of working up to the number of repetitions.

1. *Toe touching:* stand with the feet a little apart, stretch up, then touch the floor between your feet.
2. *Knee raising:* stand up, lift knees alternately, and pull them to your body with your hands.
3. *Arm swinging:* play windmills.
4. *Sit-ups:* lie on your back and sit up: as you get used to this you'll need no hands.
5. *Push-ups:* lie face down, legs straight, toes turned

under. Push yourself up with your hands. Do it any way you can to start with: eventually, your whole body will rise up in a straight line.

6. *Stationary running:* lift your feet well up off the floor, knees forward.

7. *Jumping:* up four inches, both feet together, like skipping without a rope.

Apparatus may make your exercising more impressive to your spouse, and a skipping rope or a health wheel is a modest investment; a rowing or cycling machine or a punching bag costs more for no greater benefit. All of them have the disadvantage of limiting the range of possible movements. Barbells and dumbbells capable of taking an adjustable load cannot provide as wide a variety of exercises as you can yourself, but they are more effortful for the enthusiast.

If you have had a coronary or other major health setback, graduated exercise can still be most beneficial, at the right stage and with your cardiologist's say-so. It is one way of encouraging the development of other channels, for instance, if a blood vessel has been blocked by a thrombosis. But even if you are out of condition because of ten or twenty years of sedentary living, without any specific trouble, it is wise for you to perform light, frequent exercise.

Statistically, lack of exercise is the single most important factor associated with heart attack for a man in his fifties: it is more damaging than smoking, obesity, or nervous tension.

SLEEP

"Try to get plenty of sleep" sounds like reassuring, sensible advice for anyone who hopes to live long. In fact it's a fallacy, as proved by a six-year study done by Dr. E. Cuyler Hammond, New York epidemiologist, on 900,000 men and women. About seven hours' sleep is sufficient, with ten minutes extra for men, and more is *harmful*. Among men in their fifties, for instance, those who slept nine hours a night suffered double the death rate from stroke, heart attack, or aneurysm compared with those sleeping seven hours or less. Those who slept as long as ten hours ran *four times* the risk.

The slowing down of your circulation and the horizontal position are neither of them beneficial to your heart and lungs if prolonged. Even a long flight, in which you don't move around much, is risky for your coronary circulation.

Insomnia is a boring but not killing condition, and anxiety about it is more harmful than any actual loss of sleep. If you sleep badly, check for causes for worry, take a larger daily dose of fresh air and exercise—you can spend some of your insomniac time on this—and wonder whether you are one of the many who need only about five hours' sleep at night. In any event, don't spend more than seven and a half hours in bed. Long sleep is for babies and adolescents. There's no harm, however, if you find yourself flagging part way through your day, in taking a leaf out of Churchill's book, or Truman's, and snatching a brief nap in the middle of the day.

FRESH AIR AND BREATHING

You don't have to make a thing out of breathing, but when there is an open window, or you are out of doors at some time during the day, take advantage. Have a few lung-stretching breaths, using your ribs and your diaphragm, alternately and together.

A good ploy while driving, provided you are not the driver, is to lean back in your seat, walking your hands along the roof as far as you can, and then breathing in as deeply as you can. Incidentally, this lifts your breastbone up and makes it roomy around your heart.

It is only fair to give your lungs some clean, cool, unpolluted air to breathe as often as possible. Plan your weekends and vacations accordingly.

PERSONAL AIR POLLUTION

If you live in a modern city you are breathing polluted air, tainted with gases and dangerous sulphurous particles. In the Los Angeles type of photochemical smog the action of strong sunlight on the motor-vehicle fumes makes it much worse. Your eyes sting, and it skins the lining off your lungs if you go out when it is bad.

For your health's sake you should campaign for cleaner air. But there's something a good deal simpler and more important that you can do to improve the air you breathe. The chief hazard from car exhausts is carbon monoxide, but the concentration of this gas in your blood—as carboxyhemoglobin—rarely exceeds 4 percent in the heaviest rush-hour traffic, while greater concentrations are commonplace among cigarette smokers not exposed to air pollution at all. Smoking inside your car is one of the most effective ways of getting carbon monoxide in your blood. A persistent, nasty cough, often with phlegm, and the development of chronic bronchitis are much likelier if you smoke; air pollution alone has very little effect.

THE RISKS SMOKERS RUN

Five times the normal risk of contracting disabling bronchitis: chronic bronchitis kills more than fifty thousand people a year in Britain. This risk is reduced by half in those who give up the habit.

Five times the normal risk of chest troubles after an operation.

Twenty times the normal risk of lung cancer for a heavy smoker compared with a nonsmoker. Around eight times the risk for a moderate smoker. Lung cancer kills some men in their thirties—women too. The odds slowly improve with each year after giving up smoking.

Two to three times the risk of coronary disease compared with nonsmokers. Odds worsen the more heavily you smoke; the odds are *immediately* better if you give it up.

Three times the risk of stroke if you are a smoker. Odds improve if you give it up.

Twenty times commoner in smokers is disease of the arteries to the limbs.

Peptic ulcer is commoner in smokers, and their healing is delayed. Healing is speeded at once if smoking is stopped.

Undersized babies, those with a tendency to convulsions, and those less bright (fractionally) at seven years old are commoner if the mother smoked in pregnancy.

Blood pressure is temporarily raised 10–15 millimeters of mercury by the nicotine in smoke. Cigarettes, cigarillos and cigars do the same, even if you don't inhale the latter.

Cancer of the throat and larynx are commoner in smokers, as are kidney cancer and bladder cancer.

Sinusitis, sore throats, laryngitis, and all respiratory infections are commoner in smokers; the smoke paralyzes the body's defenses.

Success in sports is less likely in smokers, especially after age twenty-five.

Ugly yellow fingers and perhaps teeth, nasty breath, irritating cough: 50 percent of all moderate smokers suffer from these.

Where nicotine comes in. Nicotine is an addictive drug like amphetamines or barbiturates. It has pleasant brain-stimulating and mood-tranquilizing effects. It also releases sugar from the liver and so peps you up this way, which may account for the desire for sweet things that sometimes grips ex-smokers in the early stages of their abstinence.

The reports published in late 1970 and early 1971 by the English Tobacco Research Council and the Royal College of Physicians in England confirm and underline what we already know about the dangers of cigarette smoking, and establish the fact that cigar tobacco, however used, is just as harmful as cigarette tobacco, or more so. It means nothing that cigar smoke is not usually inhaled: the nicotine is absorbed *in the mouth*. Nicotine increases the amount of cholesterol in the blood, and so the likelihood of thrombosis is greater. The smoke most harmful to the bronchial tubes is that of cigarillos, and it is particularly so where people have learned to use these like cigarettes. Filter tips slightly reduce bronchial irritation from smoke, but make no difference as to its cancer-producing properties; nor does a reduction in tar content matter where cancer is concerned.

NICOTINE, INHALING, AND CIGARS AND PIPES

1. *Virginian tobacco smoke* is acid and the nicotine from it cannot be absorbed through the lining of the mouth at all. Therefore, to get a satisfying dose you must inhale with your cigarettes.

2. *Cigar smoke* is alkaline and 60 percent of the nicotine in it can be absorbed through the lining of the mouth. Certainly, more would be absorbed by inhaling. Most cigar smokers do not inhale, however, and, what is more to the point, smoke only moderately.

3. *Pipe smoke* is neutral. Some of the nicotine may be absorbed through the lining of the mouth, but this will be nothing like as much as you get from inhaling a cigarette, or from inhaling on the pipe. (Pipe smokers tend to moderation, too.)

The developed nicotine addict who changes from cigarettes to cigars, cigarillos, or a pipe will always inhale to get his full quota of nicotine, and, incidentally, inhales the more harmful elements into his lungs as well. So— there's nothing to be gained by an addict changing to a different kind of smoke, although a chap who has *always* puffed a pipe or savored a cigar, almost certainly without inhaling, and in moderation, is better off, healthwise, than the average cigarette smoker.

The one cheerful note in these reports is that emphysema has been shown to be reversible. Until now, it had always been assumed that once the air sacs of the lungs were severely damaged they could never recover. This finding holds out hope for the repentant smoker even at a late stage.

According to the Chief Medical Officer in Britain, in his 1970 annual report on the State of the Public Health, smoking is the biggest single avoidable menace to health. It causes ten times as many deaths as do road accidents, and nearly as many deaths as all cancers, unrelated to smoking, put together. Smoking probably accounts for 100,000 premature deaths annually in Britain alone, and you run twice the risk of never reaching retiring age if you are a moderate smoker.

Why people smoke: It may start as something social, or as a demonstration of adulthood; it may be used as a stimulant at work; it is often used as a reaction to stress. Other strategies for coping with worries are keeping busy, food, alcohol, sex, talking with friends, or the unfashionable one (in the West) of open expression of emotion. It is wiser to sidestep stressful situations at their source, whenever possible.

Why people don't give up smoking: Whatever reason you may have had to begin smoking, if you've been a smoker for two or three years and have learned to inhale, the chances are that now you are hooked on nicotine, and go on smoking because you feel so ghastly without your drug.

Quitting: The only sensible thing to do about smoking is not to. Drugs from your doctor, chewing gum, and other aids help only psychologically: there is no substitute for will power. Prove to yourself that you are the master of your fate, not the pawn. Once you have determined to give up smoking, take the same attitude to the task as you would toward any other learning situation: you are learning to live without tobacco. You wouldn't expect instant, effortless success if you decided that you wanted to swim five miles. You'd have to try again and again before you would be able to achieve your goal. You'd *know* you'd have to work at it.

It's the same with giving up smoking: you have to *work* at it. It is hopeless to attempt to cut down gradually: this involves long-continued will power, an effort which no one can stand. If you can't plunge in at the deep end, which is best, plan your cut-down so that you can reach zero within a week. You'll feel terrible for several weeks as your brain cries out for the nicotine it's used to having, but each day the longing lessens, and ultimately it disappears. When you have got there, don't be fool enough to waste all you have been through and let yourself get hooked again.

Hang on to the rewards of giving up: improved health, increased life expectancy, and a substantial saving in money.

ALCOHOL

Alcohol has beneficial effects. You must know them: the easing of tensions; the feeling of physical warmth from the opening up of the blood vessels in the skin; immediate nourishment, since the body can burn alcohol as fuel directly; and an aid to sleep.

On the other side there is a reduction in your powers of self-criticism and a lessening of your normal inhibitions. This is how you can come to make promises—or proposals —which you regret in the morning. An occasional binge can cause acute gastritis, a headache, and a hangover, but so long as you don't fall in the river or kill yourself in a car, it isn't likely to shorten your life, unless you have a tricky heart.

What *can* be life-shortening is chronic overdrinking, leading to chronic gastritis, nerve disorders, mental deterioration, degeneration of the heart muscle, susceptibility to pneumonia, and the deadly disease of cirrhosis of the liver.

Giving up overdrinking in time can save your life.

If you are overweight you cannot afford to use alcohol because it's so high in calories.

However, if you are the right size, and healthy in lungs and heart, alcohol can be a pleasurable addition to living. Use it as a social lubricant, and, like the lubricating oil of your car, don't regard it as fuel.

TRAVEL

If you are reading this book it is a good bet that you are a person on the move, in your life and also physically, by car and plane. (Of course, if you walk it does you nothing but good.)

Driving a car can be immediately lethal if you drive carelessly, recklessly, drunkenly, nervously, or aggressively. The latter mood is enhanced by carbon monoxide in your blood. If you drive after a row with your husband or wife, when you are tired, below par in health, or merely late at night, when your brain and body are accustomed to being asleep, your efficiency at the wheel lessens. You notice less, and react slower. Various common medicines will also lower your efficiency: especially barbiturates, tranquilizers, and antidepressants; antihistamines for hay fever and other allergies; antihypertensives to control blood pressure; insulin for diabetes; isoprenaline for asthma; travel-sickness tablets; and cold cures.

The effect of a very small amount of alcohol may be dangerously heightened if you have already had some barbiturate, antihistamine, or mood-changing drug. Before you know what has hit you, you may be confused, unsteady, or sleepy, and end in a terrific crash.

Car driving can also cut you off in your prime because of the strain it imposes on the heart and arteries. The excitement of overtaking a Jaguar, or cutting into a shrinking gap between two trucks, the frustration of seeing the light turn red just as you reach it, or the stab of fear when it looks as though someone has made a miscalculation: all these raise your blood pressure, cause your heart to accelerate, and keep you in a state of fluctuating tension.

It all depends on your attitude. If you can manage to drive peaceably, this can even be a way of unwinding. One psychiatrist I know uses a long drive to relax.

Jet travel: Long flights have definite dangers: sitting cramped for five hours or more can slow the blood flow and make spontaneous clotting, as in a coronary attack or stroke, all the likelier, especially if you are eating, smoking, and drinking in transit. The tension of an air trip contributes to the situation, too, since emotion increases the coagulability of the blood. Even the most seasoned traveler gets some kind of a thrill at takeoff.

The other snag in air travel is the jangling of your circadian rhythms because of the rapid time-zone changes such travel makes possible. These rhythms are the twenty-four-hour cyclic changes in temperature, urine production, hormone manufacture, chemical processes, and electrical activity in the brain—to name a few of them. Each is controlled by a separate biological clock, and it takes at least ten days to get them all in synchronization again after flying from, say, London to San Francisco.

Out-of-phase rhythms account for the well-known jet-lag syndrome that leads businessmen to make regrettable decisions when they get down to work too soon after touchdown. A reasonable rule from this angle is: *Say what you like but sign nothing for the first forty-eight hours.* For your body's sake as well as the sake of your business, travel with a companion, and time yourself so that you will arrive at bedtime, preferably with a weekend between you and the business part of your trip. And don't overindulge, because of boredom or whatever, on the way.

SEX

This remains almost the only pleasure that isn't harmful so long as you are reasonably fit. In fact, it is a form of exercise and a first-class release from every kind of tension: the one green thing in our artificial world.

You may find that some blood-pressure medicines impair your (male) performance: this is only a temporary effect, but one reason to try the other methods for keeping your blood pressure down.

CHECK

If you were taking a trip in Apollo 16 you'd make sure that the machine on which your life depended was checked over. It would be plain common sense. You certainly need to have your body checked over for faults or possible areas of weakness that could cost you your life just as surely as a rocket misfiring in a spacecraft could.

Multiphasic screening centers—"service stations" for the human machine—have been set up in major cities all over the world.

What goes on varies from one center to another. Basically, they all give a battery of tests (available all in the same place, like the sideshows in a carnival), which combine to build up your medical profile.

The components are likely to include:

1. Your medical, personal, and environmental history, obtained either through a free-ranging interview with a physician or by a record made on a modified teaching machine. This asks questions and gives you a choice of push-button answers. If you say "Yes" to "Have you ever had pain or discomfort in your chest?" the machine will go on to find out the exact location, what makes it better or worse, and what the doctor said, if you saw him, etc.

The whole experience with the machine is like an enjoyable parlor game, and you can't lose. It holds your interest unflaggingly because it is all about you: and, of course, there's no question of criticism. In some areas, such as sex, it may be easier to be frank by touching the appropriate button than by answering a verbal or written questionnaire.

2. Your hearing.
3. Your vision.
4. Your electrocardiograph—the electrical tracing of

your heart, with analysis by consultant cardiologists, possibly computerized. Exercise EKGs may also be done, to examine how your heart behaves when extra demands are put upon it.

5. Your blood pressure.

6. Chest and abdominal X rays, with consultant reporting.

7. Measurement of your weight and size.

8. Lung-function tests to assess how efficiently your oxygenating system is working.

9. Urine tests: a check on the condition of your kidneys and urinary system and a part of your chemistry profile.

10. Blood tests, including red- and white-cell counts and microscopical examination, and your biochemical status. Measurements are made of the amount of cholesterol and other liquids in your blood—vitally important in many causes of early death—and of other such significant constituents as serum iron, uric acid, urea, calcium, and a dozen more.

11. Ladies only: Pelvic examination of reproductive organs; cervical smear; check for precancer of the womb; breast examination (clinically and by infrared mammography, also for catching precancer).

12. Other examinations, as indicated by the findings on the above, e.g., rectal examination, sigmoidoscopy, kidney X ray, breast X ray, glucose-tolerance test, etc.

The whole circus is likely to take up less than half a day, whichever sex you are. It is a method for finding your *personality-environment equation:* how you, as an individual, are standing up to the demands made upon you by your work, your home life, and your surroundings. If the equation balances, more or less, it means "don't worry": you are making the grade. If it is unstable, so is your situation, and something will crack unless adjustments are made.

The down-to-earth, positive uses of screening include:

Presymptomatic diagnosis—picking up the clues of unsuspected or incipient disease before you yourself have noticed anything wrong. This is particularly valuable where vital body systems are in danger of impairment, for instance from high blood pressure, or where there is something deadly, like cancer, in the wings.

A pointer to a change-of-life pattern, or a way of managing any disease, disability, hazardous habit, or tendency that has been revealed; for instance, if the dangerous combination of heavy smoking and a high blood cholesterol count is discovered.

A minimum standard of health by which to assess your progress, for instance your improvement in lung function if you give up smoking.

The detection of minor troubles, not in themselves important to survival, but which may well have an indirect bearing on the ultimate state of your health. These are the kinds of small, "nuisance" conditions that you might not care to bother your doctor about unless he asks, and he doesn't. For example, a smallish varicose vein could lead to a fatal hemorrhage in an accident.

Hints for working out why something may be wrong. It is the "whys" that tell how to shift into reverse gear. Coronary disease and stroke, although they can result in sudden death, are in reality parts of processes that have been going on over the years. This is what makes reversal a practical possibility once you are aware of what is happening, and why it is happening.

Screening seldom makes a complete diagnosis, but it detects the fingerprints of disease and suspicious circumstances. It identifies the vulnerable as well as those who are already victims, and for the former it is most worthwhile.

At the Institute of Directors Medical Centre in London, pioneers in the field who are now using the most modern equipment in Europe, 30 percent of all executives are found to have disorders that are diagnosed for the first time through screening; 4 percent have more than one newly discovered medical fault; 20 percent are overweight, and nearly one man in ten is seriously so—especially among the under forty-fives. It is cheering to know that between a quarter and a third of those rechecked after one year have managed to reduce. This alone must have saved some lives.

Two men and women in every ten of those who are fifty-five plus have blood pressure too high for health by any standards. In the men of under thirty-five, one in twenty-five has blood pressure higher than normal but not dangerously so—yet. There are twice as many such between thirty-five and forty-five. Women suffer less from high blood pressure before the change, but catch up soon after. Since blood pressure is often related to stress and personality interactions, environmental reconditioning—taking some of the strain off—may be all that is needed to bring the pressure down to a reasonable level. The relatively new pressure-lowering drugs may be used with effect in more obstinate cases. Lives may be saved in this way, too.

Seventeen percent are found to have very high levels of cholesterol in their blood, and as many more are on the borderline of abnormality. About a quarter of those with high blood cholesterol have sinister early changes in their heart tracings—the electrical writing on the wall. A fat-controlled diet has been shown to reverse this trend for those who take the hint.

More than one executive in ten has a definite stress illness requiring treatment, while many show milder degrees of psychological strain—revealed by the examination. These are situations to nip in the bud before they can cause harm.

One third are smoking more than eleven cigarettes a day, and taking chances with their health thereby, but some 9 percent have been able to give up smoking completely while another 22 percent are in the process of cutting down.

WHEN AND HOW OFTEN?

Although degenerative changes can start before you've lived a quarter of a century, twenty-five is a reasonable age for your first screening. If it's "all clear" at this point and you feel fine, then reexamination every two or three years should be adequate until you are forty-five. From then on, to catch trouble before it begins, your screening should become an annual duty: it should be done more often if there's a problem looming.

Medical hints for avoiding death before your time often amount to a series of prohibitions. Lord Rosenheim, President of the Royal College of Physicians, commented the other day: "I wish we could all stick by them, although it would be pretty miserable if we did. . . ."

So let us conclude this chapter with a *Nine-point Positive Life-preserving Plan for Modern Man—and His Mate*.

1. Eat wisely.
2. Exercise daily.
3. Reduce your worries, but don't delegate your physical work.
4. Ration your drinking and sleeping.
5. Travel with good sense as your companion.
6. Have your body machinery "serviced" at regular intervals.
7. Widen your outside interests.
8. Stop smoking and take no drugs without your doctor's permission.
9. Work to ease your interpersonal relations within your family, with your friends, and at work.

Heart and Arteries

In the entire history of man no plague, pestilence, or epidemic has ever seriously rivaled diseases of the heart and arteries for dealing out death. Of the 1,946,100 deaths in the United States in 1969, no fewer than 1,059,400 were due to cardiovascular disease. It's the leading cause of death in Australia, Canada, Denmark, Finland, France, the Netherlands, Norway, Sweden, Switzerland, West Germany, the United Kingdom, and the United States—all the industrialized nations of the Western world.

Fatty degeneration of the arteries—atherosclerosis—leading to heart attacks and strokes, crops up wherever life is easy and rich foods, especially fatty foods, are abundant. High blood pressure is common, exerting strains on both heart and arteries. Men of forty to fifty-five, and women just past menopause in particular, are succumbing prematurely to heart-artery disaster—many types, from tough-guy President Nasser to musician Professor Thurston Dart have died recently, and often highly trained professional people at the height of their powers are among them. Ischemic heart disease, of which coronary attacks are an expression, is affecting younger and younger men from the mid-thirties on, skimming off society's most productive citizens and cheating them of the prizes just coming within their grasp.

What is so damnable is that a large proportion of this appalling wastage—people of your caliber landing in the ashcan at their peak—could be avoided. We have the know-how to prevent it, and most of those most in danger are well able to understand and apply the principles of prevention. Yet usually they take no action until it is calamitously late. It has been proved, for instance, that you can reduce substantially your chances of having a coronary if you keep your blood cholesterol low *before* you develop symptoms. But the most stringent diet makes only a marginal difference in your prospects *after* you've had an attack. It is a weakness that runs all through our human nature. Addiction doctors find that only when a smoker has symptoms he can't ignore is he likely to be sufficiently motivated to give up the habit which intellectually he realizes may kill him.

With lung cancer, quitting smoking may still be of help. With atherosclerosis, if you wait for a warning you may never live to heed it. The infiltration of fat into your artery walls is a slow, silent, continuous process, leading inexorably to some fatal issue. To appreciate the unseen dangers and the significance of the smallest straws in the wind, you have to understand the machinery of circulation, and from this the mechanics of the Western way of death.

YOUR MACHINERY

Your heart is a four-chambered pump coupled to a system of pipes, for supplying oxygen and nutrients to the body. It also serves as a reservoir for the circulating blood. The main pumping apparatus consists of two contractile containers made of muscle, the ventricles. The right ventricle drives the blood through the lung beds to pick up oxygen and unload waste carbon dioxide from the body's combustion processes. The left ventricle has the immense task of forcing oxygenated blood along the arteries, fine-bore arterioles, and myriad minute blood vessels within the tissues all over the body, from your brain to your big toe.[1]

---

[1] For the mathematically inclined, the work done seventy times a minute by your left ventricle can be calculated this way:

$$pV + \tfrac{1}{2}mv^2 = \frac{100 \times 13.6 \times 981 \times 60}{10} + \tfrac{1}{2} \times 60 \times (50)^2 \text{ ergs}$$

when p is the mean pressure in the main artery and the output per beat is V, and the kinetic energy $\tfrac{1}{2}mv^2$ with m the mass of the blood ejected at each beat and v its velocity.

The other two chambers, the right and left atria, are collecting bags for blood returning to the heart from the lungs and the rest of the body, respectively. Valves guard the entry holes from atria to ventricles. The atria are not nearly as muscular as the ventricles, since all they have to do is push the blood directly into the latter, partly assisted by gravity. If the atria contract inefficiently or irregularly the heart is still operational. If the ventricles falter that's a heart attack.

Your heart hangs a little to the left of center in your chest, and is normally the size of its owner's bunched fist. A healthy heart isn't king-size but has first-class fuel pipes in the coronary arteries. The working heart muscle, like any other, requires a blood supply which must adjust to the work load. It is this critical supply that is directly involved in heart attacks. There are two coronary arteries, the right and the left, and there are sometimes quite extensive connections between their end branches. These can be life-saving in a disaster situation, and a way out of dangers that stop short of disaster.

In a healthy heart the muscle has no scars, nor is it degenerate with fat. Exercise will train such a heart to respond without strain to increased demands, not only by a faster rate of beating but with a greater output per beat, unlike other machines, in which efficiency falls off with faster working. A step-up in output of 500 percent presents no difficulty to a healthy heart. The arteries, too, with their strong, adjustable walls, are made to adapt to the varying needs of the muscles and organs they supply.

WHAT CAN GO WRONG

Atherosclerosis underlies all the major disasters in the heart artery system that cause premature death. It is a process that may start in the teens. Cardiologist Dr. Lawrence Lamb performed autopsies on many young American servicemen and found that in 77 percent of young men aged nineteen to twenty-two there were signs of atherosclerosis already affecting their coronary arteries. Fat compounds—lipoproteins—containing cholesterol form deposits in the walls of the arteries, including those supplying the heart muscle, the kidneys, and every other organ and tissue. These deposits may distort the vital pipelines, diminish their bore, and reduce their elasticity, thus making it harder work for the heart to drive the blood along them, and cutting down the supplies to the tissues. When atherosclerosis affects the heart's own arteries this is *coronary artery disease.*

Ischemic heart disease is the general situation of shortage of blood to the heart muscle, such as troubled President Eisenhower in his last years. His IHD was due to athero-damaged coronary arteries, as it is in most cases.

When disease of an artery severely impedes or prevents the distribution of life-giving blood to an area of tissue, that tissue dies. This is called infarction. Like ischemia, infarction can affect various organs, such as the kidneys and lungs, but if it affects the heart muscle it is called *myocardial infarction.* Infarctions that are not immediately fatal leave permanent scars, and Dr. Lamb found such scars in the hearts of some servicemen under thirty.

The fatty deposit in an artery wall may break up and extrude fragments into the artery itself, like flakes in a rusty pipe, clogging it even more. Thrombosis, the spontaneous clotting of blood inside a vessel, is likely to occur at the site of such damage to an artery wall. It is likelier, too, if there is an undue amount of fat in the blood, either temporarily or long-term. A permanently high blood cholesterol level is one of the things worth finding out about from a medical check. This level can be raised temporarily, after a fatty meal, or because of emotion. Dr. Malcolm Carruthers, working with racing drivers, found their blood plasma milky white with fat compounds released under the influence of the excitement hormone, adrenaline.

Spontaneous clotting in a coronary artery is called coronary *thrombosis,* and the result is myocardial infarction. Thrombosis can be a dramatic event if there is rapid, complete blockage of a major branch of a coronary artery, or infarction may happen silently, with the gradual occlusion of a vessel.

Atherosclerosis itself is a generalized disorder which can affect various parts of the blood-transport system to a varying extent. It is responsible for many of the conditions that we usually attribute to increasing age, for instance the drop-off in athletic prowess, the dimming of sight and memory. But however deadly its end results, atherosclerosis is a very gradual process, commonly taking thirty years to reach a danger point. The highly dangerous acute stage lasts about a month and is marked by myocardial infarction coming on with a coronary attack, perhaps preceded briefly by angina, or by the less alarming development of angina alone.

Fifty percent of men die within three months of their first coronary attack, most within the month. But if you weather the first storm you have a second chance of living a reasonable span. Your heart can compensate for the loss of one coronary artery if there is a good series of connections between what is left—collateral circulation—and if these are encouraged to develop by careful, graduated exercise, at the right time.

Temporary shortage of blood to any muscle that you are using causes pain, like the pain in your legs that you get if you go on and on running. Sometimes, while a blood supply is adequate for normal use, it is not enough to cope with any additional load. Atherosclerosis of the arteries to the legs, Buerger's disease, can cause intermittent limping and leg pain on walking, which is relieved by standing still for a few minutes. If it is the heart muscle that is affected, the extra work involved in walking uphill, or after a meal, may lead to cramplike pains in the chest, sometimes extending to the jaw, abdomen, or arms.

Angina pectoris is the name of this kind of heart pain, and although it is usually brought on by physical effort, emotion alone may precipitate it, even in a dream. A rare form, *tobacco angina,* is brought on by smoking. Angina may be the forerunner of coronary attack, as it was for a year with journalist Cyril Watling,[1] or it may continue for many otherwise uneventful years. Unpredictability is characteristic of atherosclerotic disease.

Coronary spasm occurs when fatty deposits cause the muscle fibers in the arterial walls to squeeze tight temporarily, thus reducing the blood flow through them. This may produce angina-type pain lasting longer than the few minutes of an ordinary anginal attack, but it is less serious than coronary thrombosis.

Atherosclerosis of the aorta, the main artery leading from the heart, may result in a tear between the layers of its wall; the weak place that bulges may ultimately give way. This is an *aortic aneurysm,* something that may sometimes be successfully repaired with Teflon tubing, but is far safer avoided.

Hypertension is the Greek for high (blood) pressure. You have to have some blood pressure to live. If your blood pressure suddenly falls, from psychic shock or loss of blood, or when you get up from a warm bed too quickly and pass water, you may faint. What makes it high is a natural tendency, much as some people are taller than others. The trouble with hypertension is that it puts a permanent strain on the heart, increases atherosclerosis, and makes a coronary or a stroke more likely. A dangerously high blood pressure is likely to crop out in the un-

---

[1] *Don't Be Afraid of a Coronary,* 1970.

lucky ones between forty-five and sixty, but usually, in these people, it has been above average by forty or less. A woman who had higher than average blood pressure when she was pregnant is likely at fifty to have symptoms of disease.

As with any other muscle, increased work makes the heart grow bigger, especially the ventricle that is taking the main load. In high blood pressure it is the left ventricle that takes the rap. It is fine for a muscle like your biceps to bulge like a grapefruit, but for a muscle that is a hollow ball, enlargement means it operates less efficiently. If you have a relatively thin rubber bulb, you can squeeze it to pump out air or fluid, as with the doctor's syringe for washing wax from your ears. On the other hand, if the rubber is very thick, it is difficult to push out the full contents. Another snag in the enlarged heart of high blood pressure is that there may be just too much of it for the coronary arteries to fuel: this is one cause of myocardial ischemia.

Arteriosclerosis is the condition in which the arteries have become stiff and fragile because of the deposit of calcium in the fatty plaques of atherosclerosis. The result may be a progressive shutting down of many of the arteries to the brain; this happens to some middle-aged, but to more old, people. *Stroke* implies a sudden disaster, comparable with a coronary, but tending to come a little later in life. It is usually the result of a raised blood pressure proving to be too much of a strain for a weakened, brittle, atherosclerotic artery. A damaged area in the wall may give way, and escaping blood cause more or less havoc in the soft brain tissue. The famous surgeon John Hunter said that his life lay at the mercy of any rogue who chose to enrage him: he did, in fact, die in a fit of anger from the kind of stroke called *cerebral hemorrhage*.

Cerebral thrombosis is spontaneous clotting in a brain artery. It usually comes on more gradually than cerebral hemorrhage, but is also due, basically, to atherosclerosis. *Cerebral embolism,* the third type of stroke, is the blocking of an artery by a piece from a clot dislodged from some other part of the body. This disaster has the most sudden onset of all. It can follow from a coronary thrombosis if the clot extends into the heart itself—as if one major calamity were not enough.

Sometimes an artery supplying the lungs is blocked: this is called *pulmonary embolism*. Clotting in the deep veins of the leg, for instance, may occur after an operation, in pregnancy, or on the pill, or when you keep unnaturally immobile on a long journey. A detached fragment from the clot may lodge in a lung artery, making useless the area of tissue it supplied. Sometimes the clotting may take place directly in the lung artery, as in a coronary artery.

Damage or disease of the lungs reduces their oxygenating efficiency and makes it necessary for both sides of the heart to work harder, to allow the various organs to get enough oxygen to function. Disorders such as emphysema make it tougher to pump blood through the lung tissue, and put a strain mainly on the right ventricle, which enlarges. Other disorders that jeopardize the heart's efficiency include congenital defects, rheumatic disorders such as mitral stenosis (stiffening of the valve between the right atrium and its ventricle), and bacterial endocarditis (infection within the heart). Better living conditions and antibiotics have made both of these latter troubles less common and less dangerous.

The actual muscle of the heart may be substandard, due to damage from infarction, fatty infiltration between the fibers, or alcoholic degeneration, the latter a cause that is on the increase.

These are the ways in which your heart and arteries may let you down. *Are you a particular risk?*

PREDISPOSING FACTORS TO HEART/ARTERY DISEASE

You should worry about atherosclerosis, the daddy of them all, if:

1. You are *overweight*. You stand a better chance with your arteries if you are slightly under the average for your height and sex.

2. One or both of your parents is dead. Particularly if there is a hereditary tendency to high blood pressure in the family.

3. You have more than 270 milligrams percent cholesterol in your blood: this constitutes a risk of coronary attack, plus, by 300 percent.

4. You are male (or a female over fifty, no longer protected by your sex hormones).

5. You are basically thick-set.

6. You exercise little or irregularly: this increases the risk of a coronary by 300 percent.

7. You own one or more cars, radios, TV sets.

8. You smoke plenty of *cigarettes*, cigarillos, or cigars. Ten a day doubles your chances of infarction, more than twenty nearly quadruples it. Angina is not so closely associated with smoking as the real disasters are.

9. You are ambitious, restless, full of drive, aggressive, conscientious, and energetic; you control your impulses and pride yourself on dependability and getting things done. Such a *personality* correlates with high blood cholesterol, and increases your coronary risk to six times the standard.

10. You are often stressed, anxious, angry, excited. You overwork. This raises your blood pressure and revs up your heart rate "while you wait." A car driver's pulse rate is frequently 150 per minute in traffic, and in Apollo 14 the astronauts' heart rates quadrupled at the first setback.

11. You drink plenty of alcohol. Its weakening effect on the heart muscle may be the final straw in a chancy situation.

12. Your *blood pressure is raised* appreciably above the norm for your age. This in turn causes more atheromatous deposits in your arteries.

13. You fly long distances, drinking, eating, dozing, and worrying about your business all the way.

14. You cut out vacations as inessential, or you combine them with a business trip.

15. You scrap with your wife/husband/life partner.

16. You are on the pill or pregnant, which increases your thrombotic tendency.

17. You work with someone who needles you.

18. You have a one-child family (how this can help to multiply your responsibilities I wouldn't hazard a a guess).

19. You frequently feel a sense of exhaustion.

Note: The four most significant factors are overweight, cigarette smoking, personality, and raised blood pressure. Blood pressure is measured by an instrument known as a sphygmomanometer, consisting of an inflatable cuff to go around your upper arm and a pressure gauge. It is expressed by a double reading, say 120/70. The first figure represents the systolic pressure in millimeters of mercury, that is, when the ventricles are actually contracting to drive the blood out. The second, lower, is the diastolic pressure, when the ventricles are relaxing. Blood pressure varies with age, increasing through childhood and onward, and also with your minute-to-minute activity and emotional state, but a consistent systolic reading of 150 in a man of under fifty is definitely above normal, and one of 180 at any age doubles the standard risk of a coronary or a stroke.

One or more of these predisposing factors places you in the athero-prone group, with a fair likelihood of joining the coronary class, and indicates that you need preventive treatment, in the same way as children have the routine immunization against polio. Don't be disappointed to find yourself in the risk set. You wouldn't really like to be the type least likely to get a coronary. According to the distilled wisdom of a British Medical Association congress on the subject, the lowest risk subject is apparently: "An effeminate municipal worker or embalmer, completely lacking in physical or mental alertness, without drive, ambition or competitive spirit, who has never attempted to meet a deadline of any kind.

"A man of poor appetite, subsisting on fruits and vegetables, laced with corn or whale oil. Detesting tobacco and spurning ownership of radio, television or motor car. He has a full head of hair and is swarthy and unathletic in appearance, yet he is constantly straining his puny muscles in exercise. He is low in income, blood sugar, uric acid, and cholesterol. He has been on nicotinic acid, pyridoxine, and a long-term anticoagulant ever since his prophylactic castration."

If this isn't you, read on:

PRE-ACTION

The important thing is to begin soon enough. A polio shot isn't of any use after the virus is in your system. Similarly, with heart or artery disease it works the same way. Atherosclerosis, before the acute stage is reached, may well be reversible or at least capable of being halted, but a myocardial infarct leaves a permanently damaged heart, however you alter your *modus vivendi*. Thirty-five is a suitable age to go in for prevention, if you've already missed the twenty-five mark. Besides, you are likely to have some sense and solidity of purpose by that age.

You can't change your parents, nor the heredity and body build they landed you with, but you can take note of warnings and protect yourself from cardiovascular demise by reversing other risk factors. This involves a program of exercise and general physical activity, attention to your diet and nutritional status (as described in the last chapter), and a review of your living pattern and habits for dangerous flaws.

SPECIFICALLY

1. Get your weight down to just below what it should be: Keep it there (See Chapter IV).
2. If you are a male, make the most of it. If you are a female approaching the menopause, discuss with

your doctor the advisability of hormone-replacement treatment.

3. Exercise regularly. Especially, *walk*.
4. *Keep your blood cholesterol within low, healthy limits,* not more than 270 milligrams percent, by not eating to excess, particularly of those foods rich in ready-made cholesterol. A four-year study just completed by the New York Coronary Club showed that people on a diet low in saturated fats —i.e., those containing cholesterol—had a marked lowering of their blood cholesterol level, and just one third the incidence of coronary attacks of a control group eating normally.

It may be that all you need do to keep your blood cholesterol at a safe level is to cut off the fat from your meat, avoid pastry, sausages, and cream, spread your butter thinly, and avoid eating too much egg yolk, liver, or sweetbreads. Since ingesting polyunsaturated fats helps lower the blood cholesterol, include in your diet cooking oils, such as sunflower or corn oil, and soft, polyunsaturated margarines. Eat as you please of lean meat, fish, fruit, and vegetables.

If your doctor thinks you ought to avoid saturated fats completely, try this diet:

BREAKFAST
Fresh fruit, grapefruit, stewed apples or prunes.
Toast or rolls.
Margarine high in polyunsaturates.
Marmalade, jam, or honey.
Tea or coffee with fat-free milk. Sugar as liked.

MIDMORNING
Tea or coffee with fat-free milk, or fruit juice.
Plain cracker.

LUNCH
Lean meat or fish, 30 grams.
Potatoes, boiled or cooked with vegetable oil.

Any other vegetable.
Milk pudding made with fat-free milk.
Fresh, stewed, or canned fruit. Coffee.

MIDAFTERNOON

Bread, Ry-Krisp, or toast.
Polyunsaturated margarine, jam, syrup, honey.
Plain cracker, or cake made with margarine and no
  egg.

SUPPER

As lunch.

Vegetable oils, e.g., corn oil, to be used for
cooking throughout.

Allowed unlimitedly: Vegetables, fruits, margarine, bread, white fish.

Not allowed at all: Brains, eggs, liver, bacon, butter, sweetbreads, tripe, veal, cheese, cream, and
milk.

Suitable for main dish: Lamb, chicken, turkey,
cod, halibut.

Your doctor may suggest that you take tablets
rather than conform to a rigid diet to reduce your
blood cholesterol. There are two types: cholestyra-
mine, which traps cholesterol in your intestines so
that you don't absorb it; and clofibrate (Atro-
mid-S), which prevents the body from synthesizing
the stuff. The latter is pleasanter to take, and more
frequently effective—in 75 to 80 percent of people—but even so, you may dislike the thought of
taking a tablet on a permanent daily basis. Women,
however, do the same thing for years with the pill.
For them, clofibrate may be helpful after menopause; for a man with a tendency to high cholesterol, he may take this medication from thirty
to about seventy.

5. Stop silting up your lungs and endangering your
   coronary circulation by smoking. This habit has
   also a positive correlation with high blood cho-

lesterol. Cure yourself of the addiction, but expect a rough two weeks while you do it. Don't fool yourself by switching to filter tips, cigarillos, cigars, or a pipe. If you've been a cigarette addict you'll manage to inhale efficiently enough with whatever you smoke to get your dose of nicotine—and be little better off.

6. Drink if it relaxes you, and if you can manage moderation, i.e., not more than two before dinner.

7. Take two months off if you are a woman on the pill. Use some other method of contraception during that period.

8. Drive quietly and peaceably and avoid long flights as much as possible.

9. Don't be so materially minded.

10. Get your blood pressure, blood cholesterol, and EKG checked regularly; weigh yourself regularly.

And finally: change your philosophy to something gentler. Professor Jeremy Morris, leading British research worker in the field of hypertension and heart disease, has said that the original hippie philosophy in San Francisco had a good deal to recommend it for those who wanted to avoid a coronary. Find out your own best tempo and the amount of challenge that stimulates you but stops short of stress. When you are under strain try to get the support and relief you need—a psychiatrist might help.

Find out what relaxes you and practice it. Winston Churchill's secret, or one of them, was sleep: not long, dangerous lying in overnight, but the one-hour nap in the middle of the day, and the habit of catnapping when there was nothing else useful to be done, e.g., during someone else's speech.

Never take it for granted that people understand each other; a great deal of unnecessary strain originates in faulty communication.

Live more in the present, and be less concerned with mistakes in the past and fears for the future. Peace of mind is for today.

Profits, promotion, prestige, and other forms of personal accomplishment may need reevaluation. Don't race with the rats. Live instead, and cultivate secondary interests even if your work is absorbing. The right philosophy for you is probably the greatest in terms of protection from heart trouble. The go-getter's risk of coronary trouble or other artery failure is far more than that of the easy rider, regardless of age, blood cholesterol, etc.

Determine what you have left to live for, apart from keeping your heart happy: the threefold pleasures of wine, women, and entertainment—be it music, art, theater, cards, or sports; athletics of all sorts, so long as you train for them; collecting; creative pleasures, from carpentry to playing Beethoven; mastering a new subject, from Yiddish to Cordon Bleu cookery; cultivating a garden, or, more profitably, your friendships.

YELLOW WARNING

You could be on the low road to disaster if you find from a screening that you have high blood cholesterol, high blood pressure, or something wrong with your EKG. Your physician will give you the guidelines to getting onto the right path. If you smoke, overdrink, or are overweight, you know what to do without his telling you, but his personal concern may help.

These are also certain symptoms to watch out for:

Breathlessness on exertion may indicate that you are out of condition, overweight, anxious; that you have a respiratory condition, ranging from a cold to chronic bronchitis; or that your heart is feeling the strain. Let your doctor listen to it, and then listen to him.

Irritability, nervousness, loss of energy and of the power of concentration, and insomnia could all be early indications of high blood pressure, but are even more likely to be due to mental strain and anxiety.

Headaches and dizziness are occasionally later symptoms of high blood pressure but again they may merely reflect worry. Find out which, through your doctor.

Chest pain that comes on after walking, after meals, or when you are upset may be due to angina. If so, it is usually of a pressing, constricting nature, though some people simply describe it as "sharp." It is commonly felt behind the upper part of the breast bone, but may extend to the neck, jaw, back, arms, or upper abdomen. Often you want to belch with it, and for this reason it may be mistaken for indigestion. Of course such a pain may indeed be caused by trouble in the digestive system, or by anxiety. The chest pain of anxiety, however, is usually a dull, persistent ache below the left-breast area, maybe lasting for hours. The pain of angina rarely goes on for more than three minutes.

Very severe, crushing chest pain may be the result of coronary spasm or incipient thrombosis.

Nosebleeds may result from an infection in the nose or from a vessel that happens to be weak. It may also be a sign that your blood pressure is somewhat up or that the vessels have weakened walls.

Yellow lumps—xanthelasma—just under the skin of the eyelids indicate a high blood cholesterol level. A low-cholesterol diet and other means of reducing the blood cholesterol often succeed in making these disappear—a good sign.

Blue color and perhaps congested veins in your neck are certain signs that you should see a doctor about your heart.

Palpitation or irregularity of heart beats can be due to trouble in the heart but is more often associated with dyspepsia, nervous conditions, or as a reaction to alcohol, tobacco, caffeine in coffee or tea, a heavy meal, or excitement.

Fatigue for little or no reason: this may mean nothing, or something.

If you are experiencing any of these could-be warning symptoms, find out why, from your physician. No book is a substitute for a personal consultation with an expert. And remember, as you follow his advice, that overwork, worry, and emotional stress are just as harmful as sudden or prolonged physical exertion among the precipitating causes of breathlessness and a feeling of exhaustion.

THE CRUNCH

The sooner you try to live a healthy life, the safer you are. If you dally indefinitely you may die for it. If the crunch comes and you survive the first assault, you have a second chance. But this time it will be harder, require all your strength of character, and be slower to show results.

Let's consider a handful of the lucky ones, people who went through their worst experiences several years ago, took warning, and are now back in circulation, wiser but not sadder men and women.

EDWIN T.: ANGINA PECTORIS

Edwin was a fattish man of forty-five who ran a successful dress business in London's Oxford Street. Every day, for his health's sake, he'd walk across Hyde Park to and from his lunch, at one of the restaurants by the Serpentine. Once or twice, after a particularly good lunch or one which had been the setting for an important business deal, he noticed an odd twinge of pain in his chest on the return trip.

It became more frequent—every day—except on Sundays, when it was his habit to read the papers in a relaxed fashion after his midday meal. His wife thought he had businessman's ulcers, and in the end persuaded him to see a doctor. But, as Dr. Guido Pincherle of the Institute of Directors Medical Centre has recently pointed out, businessmen get peptic ulcers *less than half* as commonly as average. It's the businessman's heart, not his stomach, that gives under the strain.

So although the doctor's questions ranged over other possibilities, he was concerned about the character of the pain—was it bursting or pressing?—and also about what brought it on. Anginal pain is most easily provoked after a meal; with walking, particularly the first walk of the day, or the first hole of golf (first-effort angina), with emotion; on stooping, but more often on lying down, which puts the heart at a disadvantage. One boxer was regularly awakened by anginal pain because he dreamed of his old fights. Typically, anginal pain lasts only a few minutes, and Edwin found that his stopped if he stood still for two or three minutes.

Physical examination cannot establish with certainty the diagnosis of angina pectoris, but an EKG after exercise (radio-recorded *during* exercise is even better) showed that the blood supply to Edwin's heart fell short in such circumstances: he had cardiac ischemia, the basis of angina pectoris. The commonest reason for this is the silting of the coronary arteries with atherosclerosis, but there may also be remediable causes such as anemia and thyroid disorder, and contributory factors such as high blood pressure, diabetes, and obesity.

Thorough examination revealed that in addition to his fat surplus, Edwin's hemoglobin was slightly subpar, and he had a mild diabetic tendency. His blood pressure was no worry, and he did not smoke, but clearly, his eating habits could do with correction. He increased the iron-containing foods: liver, bran, sardines, corned beef, cocoa, and green vegetables, while decreasing the overall quantity of food, particularly sweets and other carbohydrates.

In daily life, he had to adjust to his disability by avoiding large meals, walks in the cold wind, sudden strenuous activity, or going to bed in a cold room. He applied himself to a course of coronary training, gradually increasing the length of his gentle, daily walk. He brought his wife into his business as an equal partner, which halved his load of responsibility and improved their relationship at a time when it was growing stale. He began to take pleasure in his grandchild.

The only medicine that Edwin used was trinitrate tablets. These dilate the coronary arteries, if they are healthy enough, but also enable the heart to operate more economically. They act best if chewed up in the mouth, but not swallowed: absorption is faster through the lining of the mouth than through the stomach. Trinitrate acts if taken just before or during an attack, but long-acting nitrates don't reduce the likelihood of attacks. Edwin did not use the latter.

Edwin died recently, exactly forty-four years after his first severe attack of angina, an example of the way in which simple measures, applied consistently, can turn the tide. Nowadays there are other drug treatments available. Practolol decreases the heart's response to stimulation and reduces the number of anginal attacks; clofibrate may help clear the coronary arteries of deposits; and chlorpropamide stimulates the natural production of insulin in mild diabetes. But a better end result could hardly be expected.

THELMA L.: HYPERTENSION

Thelma L. was fifty-two. Her blood pressure had gone up during her two pregnancies and had remained on the high side of the normal range afterward: 140/80. However, it wasn't until after her menopause at the age of forty-eight that she began to have symptoms of loss of energy, irritability, and unreasonableness. Her family put them down to "her age." The development of hypertensive heart trouble in her sister, some nine years older, did not strike them as significant at the time. Two events in her fifty-third year shook Thelma's confidence. One she kept to herself and worried over in private: an episode of blood in her urine, with no other symptom. The other was the sudden, painless, but lurid-looking appearance of a bloodshot eye. A small vessel in the white conjunctiva had broken spontaneously, of no importance in itself. However, it made her go to her doctor and in turn directed his attention to her blood pressure, which he found substantially raised. The palpitations which she had noticed recently he considered merely symptoms of her natural anxiety about her health.

Already her heart had begun to enlarge so as to withstand the pressure, and she had noticed that the walk up a nearby hill left her breathless as it never used to. Of course, she was heavier and less active than she had been as a young mother. Her life expectancy, without treatment, would have been unpleasantly short.

Thelma's life-saving course included the reduction of, and support in, anxieties and stresses, which she—like most of us—had; the reassuring knowledge that her blood pressure was being treated and that her health was in expert hands; and the cooperation of her rather thoughtless family of an academic husband and two adolescent sons. Some measure of weight reduction was beneficial, and she was able to achieve this with her good sense and restraint.

For its own mildly lowering effect on the blood pressure, and because it enabled her to respond to safer, smaller doses of the drugs prescribed by her doctor, Thelma took steps to reduce her salt intake moderately.

She avoided ham, bacon, Spam, sausages, meat and fish paste, canned and smoked fish, meat extracts, canned vegetables, bottled sauces, pickles and dressings, cheese, water biscuits, cream crackers, malted milk, and chocolate beverages. She added no salt at the table, and restricted her daily margarine to an ounce, her milk to a pint.

She freely ate fruit, fruit juices, jam and honey, fresh and frozen vegetables, boiled rice and spaghetti, pepper, herbs, mustard, spices, and curry powder for flavoring.

The hypotensive (pressure-lowering) drug chosen by Thelma's doctor was methyl-dopa, which has the particular advantage of reducing the pressure whether the patient is standing or lying down, while the other types only work when he is erect; the side effect of lassitude wore off as she continued the treatment. She also took a diuretic to help rid her of excess fluid.

Thelma is sixty-two now, slimmer and fitter than she was ten years ago, and her EKG and heart size show improvement. The development of complications, including the deadliest—coronary attack, heart or kidney failure, and stroke—has been held off by blood pressure control. Any man or woman of under sixty who has a diastolic blood pressure of 105 or more probably ought to receive pressure-lowering treatment—*for life*. The outlook for a

woman with high blood pressure is rather better than it is
for a man, but men tend to have fewer side effects from
the drugs used.

Thelma smoked only on rare social occasions, but had
she been anything of a smoker it would have been man-
datory for her to give it up.

TOBY: CORONARY THROMBOSIS

Toby was a lawyer of some repute, constantly in demand and all over the place, spending his days on his toes
in court and half his nights working on his briefs. He
smoked like a machine as he worked, using at least forty
cigarettes a day. When he was pressed for time—a chronic
condition with Toby—he would take a couple of drinks
instead of stopping for a meal. He had a reputation for
always being on the ball, was never ill, and was slim as a
whippet. He had an eventful social life and two women,
one his wife and the other a reporter who often wrote up
his cases.

He was obsessed with making a name for himself and
success was very near. He was thirty-eight. Once or twice
he'd had odd pains which, on looking back, could have
been anginal, but he was utterly unprepared for the crash.
He had had a particularly hectic week and had just won
a big case that had been going on for some time. He
decided to spend a quiet evening at his mistress Angela's
place to recuperate. She whipped him up a simple meal—
an omelet, as a matter of fact, rich in cholesterol—and
he sat, luxuriating, while she cleared the table. The telephone jangled—it might be his wife.

That's when it gripped him: pains like red-hot wires
boring and twisting in his chest, shooting down his arms,
through to his back, up into his neck. He was cold, sweating, nauseated . . . Angela came through to see who was
on the phone, took one look at Toby, and sized the situation up. Toby had only the haziest impression of what
happened after this but he remembered the waves of pain
receding after a morphine injection from a strange doctor,
the ride to the hospital in an ambulance, and a nurse with

cool hands telling him to keep still, that he was over the worst: as indeed he was. Eighty-one percent of those who die with their first coronary do so during the first hour and it makes very little difference whether they are in the hospital under intensive care or at home. Every hour that passes after the first made it less likely that Toby would be one of the 1500 who die of a coronary every day in the United States.

It used to be the fashion to keep a coronary victim lying at attention in bed for weeks while a nurse poured soup into his mouth. Toby was allowed to sit up as soon as he felt inclined, and he was out in a chair two days later. Thrombosis in the veins, which used to be a problem with such immobilized patients, no longer is. Nevertheless, for the first month his life hung in the balance, and it was reassuring that his heart was being monitored and that resuscitating apparatus and skill were at hand, including a defibrillator to get his heart back on the beat if it started contracting irregularly.

For six weeks Toby's activity was minimal, except for mental activity. He put his lawyer's mind to the evidence. What had caused this near miss—and could it cause another attack:

Obesity—No.
Cigarettes—Yes.
Sex—Yes (he was the wrong one).
Occupation—Yes.
Mental stress—Yes: in work and women.
Body build—No.
Blood pressure ⎫
Blood cholesterol ⎬—Not checked before this.
EKG ⎭
Exercise—Patchy.
Ambition, drive, restlessness—In excess.

For three months more Toby concentrated on living again, and working out a way to continue the process. *Smoking* was a mustn't; with the only too genuine threat of death to spur him on he didn't find giving it up too difficult. *Diet:* Anything that might reverse atherosclerosis was worth trying, so he set himself to acquiring a taste for a low-cholesterol diet, high in polyunsaturates. *Exercise* was a chancy one: he remembered friends who had killed themselves by foolhardy activities before they had had time or training to develop a collateral circulation. The most dangerous form of exercise for Toby would have been to try to push his car in a snowdrift: heavy work in the cold, his mood laced with anger and frustration would be deadly. Toby, in due course, took up horseback riding, an uncompetitive sport that suited his new image.

The big change in Toby's life, however, was his attitude. A cooler, more intellectual approach to his cases brought him no diminution of success and respect. Careful avoidance of stress-making situations and people likely to engender steam was as important as his own attitude. When he cannot avoid an encounter with someone who needles him, he takes a tranquilizer in advance. He has sorted out his marital tensions too. He and Angela have been married nearly ten years now, for this whole frightening affair happened back in 1961.

Toby is perhaps not as rich as he might have been, but he would rather live with a slightly lower income than die a millionaire. His doctor, of course, keeps close watch on him.

Some medicines have helped Toby survive, including a year and a half of anticoagulants, but basically this has been a personal victory for Toby, and a lucky one. Heroic operations to unblock occluded coronary arteries have been tried and research is concentrating on these small but vital vessels, but there's no easy answer yet.

6

Lungs and Breathing Apparatus

Breath is life. A continuous supply of oxygen is essential to the functioning of every cell of every tissue, yet the body has almost no storage capacity for the stuff. This means that if you stop breathing for as long as three minutes you will probably have suffered irreparable harm to your brain, that most complex, delicate, and personal of organs.

Gasping or struggling for breath uses up what oxygen there is in the body all the quicker, and even if your breathing is restored a few minutes later, the damage will have been done, unless somehow a supply of oxygen has been kept up in your lungs.

EMERGENCY

It could happen to anyone. It could happen to you—respiratory arrest from carbon monoxide poisoning (e.g., car exhaust); a coronary; electric shock; drowning. If it happened to you, you couldn't do a thing to save yourself, although the slightest delay would mean curtains. So it is a sensible precaution if everyone in the family has a clear idea of what to do if anyone stops breathing; and if up-to-date illustrated instructions about resuscitation, reading something like this, are kept immediately available.

KISS OF LIFE

Place the victim on his back.

Kneel by him and bend his head back, then hold his jaw up with one hand.

Quickly hook out any debris or dentures from his mouth with the other hand.

Pinch his nose and keep it pinched.

Take a deep breath, put your mouth over his mouth, and blow steadily until you see his chest rise.

Quickly remove your mouth to let the victim exhale passively.

Repeat ten times a minute.

Between breaths, call for help.

If air enters the stomach it will bulge visibly; push the air out by pressing on the abdomen.

This highly efficient, on-the-spot method of artificial respiration was first described some time ago, by a gentleman named Elisha (II Kings 4:34), and rediscovered in 1957. It has the tremendous advantage of requiring no apparatus and of being capable of application, as necessary, in almost any situation, even in water, before the drowning person has been brought to land. It is, incidentally, pointless to think of emptying the lungs of water before the kiss: seconds count.

If, despite the kiss, breathing does not start in two or three minutes, and someone else is on the scene, try *heart massage*—as well as, but not instead of, the kiss, which must continue while there is any hope of revival.

The victim must lie on a firm surface. Alternately apply pressure and relaxation with the heel of your hand between the middle and lower thirds of his breastbone, at a rate of eighty per minute.

This may do for the heart what the kiss of life does for the lungs: keep up some sort of output while the natural function has a chance to begin again.

In carbon monoxide poisoning and salt water drowning, it is primarily the breathing that fails. In heart attack, electric shock, and fresh water drowning, death is due primarily to the stopping of the heart, but both massage and artificial respiration are likely to be required.

If you can keep all systems going—after a fashion—until professional help arrives, there's a good chance for survival. The kiss can save a life in the direct disaster, and you don't need to know much to apply it. But for dealing with the commoner, drawn-out dangers, it is useful to understand the working of:

YOUR OXYGENATING PLANT

It consists of an entry chamber, the nose, which warms, humidifies, and, to a certain extent, filters the air you breathe in. The warming is undoubtedly effective, since air that goes into the front of the nose at 43° F. has been heated to 86° by the time it reaches the back. Like an iceberg, the visible part of the nose is much smaller than the part you can't see.

It leads the processed air to the entrance to the windpipe, or trachea, a circular tube held in shape by rings of cartilage, so that you can turn your head from side to side without kinking it. Try swallowing while you are looking over your shoulder—it's uncomfortable. But breathing is no problem. A lid closes over the top of the windpipe while you swallow, and you choke if it is not quite shut in time. A cough forcibly bursts open this lid with an uprush of air.

The trachea travels down through the neck to divide into the two main airways into the lungs, the right and left bronchial tubes. The right-hand pipe runs more directly downward, so that if you inhale a peanut, it is likely to lodge on this side. The bronchi divide and subdivide into smaller and smaller bronchioles, ending ultimately in millions of gossamer-thin air sacs. Each is covered with a tracery of the most delicate blood vessels, and it is here that the vital exchange of gases takes place, between blood and air.

The blood takes on fresh oxygen and gives up used carbon dioxide as it streams over the air sacs, whose combined surface totals between twenty-three and twenty-six feet. This is the essence of respiration, the purpose of the whole system. The intimately involved networks of air passages and blood vessels comprise the lungs, each enclosed in a double bag of membrane called the pleura. The heart lies between the two lungs. Around them all is the cage of ribs, muscle alternating with bones, and below, a great sheet of muscle, the diaphragm, which separates chest from abdomen.

The lungs have no power of their own, but passively follow the movements of the chest wall and diaphragm. To accomplish the indrawing of breath the diaphragm moves downward and the ribs space out from each other. Either the ribs or the diaphragm alone can operate the system, but normally the latter is responsible for three quarters of the work, especially in men. To breathe out, the ribs close on each other and the diaphragm rises to compress the lungs, but in the ordinary way this is mainly a matter of relaxation, and little effort is involved.

The human breathing system is an ingenious adaptation of the air bladder used as a buoyancy device in our fishier ancestors. It has the same disadvantage as a London bus: exit and entry must take place through the same passage. This allows only a partial exchange of air at each breath— five sixths remains. However, within its limits the apparatus works quite effectively. Refinements include muscle in the walls of the bronchial tubes, particularly the smaller ones, to alter the air flow, and mucus-producing glands to help in keeping them from silting up. From the bronchioles to the back areas of the nose the breathing passages have a special lining. The free border of each cell bears hundreds of tiny, hairlike processes, whose continuous task is to waft mucus, with debris and bacteria entangled in it, like a moving staircase up to the main exit. There it can be cleared by coughing or quietly swallowing.

The importance of the cleansing system can be judged by the fact that some twenty billion particles of foreign matter are breathed into the lungs every day by a city resident. The movement of the cell hairs is automatic and autonomous, and continues even for a while after death. Cigarette smoke or radiation stop them cold.

The normal rate of breathing is twelve to twenty times a minute for a relaxed adult, but this and the depth of the breaths can adjust to supply fifteen to twenty times more on demand. Panting brings in twenty gallons of air per minute.

The breathing center in the brain acts as a computer by receiving information from other parts of the brain, from the muscles and tissues via the nerves, and from the blood, by chemical changes in it, thus calculating the requirement for ventilation, i.e., breathing. A buildup of carbon dioxide in your blood, for instance, gives you an unpleasant, weak feeling and automatically starts you panting. Fever and exercise also induce faster breathing, quite apart from the effects of carbon dioxide. Failure of the heart, partial or complete, has a similar result.

You can alter the rate and depth of your breathing at will, or even hold your breath, but normally the robot pilot is in charge, and breathing, like other natural phenomena, runs to a rhythm.

A cough is an explosion set off by irritation in the breath tubes, and useful for ridding them of rubbish or infected matter. A snag here is that congestion, for any reason, or a cancer, may also cause irritation and the cough response—to no purpose. A sneeze is an explosion released through the nose, and triggered by irritation of its lining. It may have enough force to propel particles as far as twenty feet. It may be set off as well by hay fever, for instance, as by infected material in the nose. Laughter and crying both consist of deep breaths in, then short spasmodic jerks of the diaphragm, usually when it has been irritated on the abdominal side; and a yawn is a ridiculous, highly infectious, huge breath with the mouth wide open —which achieves nothing, as far as we know.

WHAT CAN GO WRONG

Minor troubles in the upper reaches of the respiratory system are commonplace, and your body can ride them out. The universal cold in the head, for instance, doesn't usually prevent you from going about your normal business, or even from meeting the extra demands of some sport. But if a large area of the lungs themselves is compromised, this spells danger to your life. It can happen in lung cancer, bronchitis, emphysema, asthma, pulmonary infarction, and, acutely, in pneumonia. It used to happen with TB, but the dangers of this disease, like those of pneumonia, have been largely abated by modern antibiotics. Coughing up blood, the dramatic symptom that used to indicate the desperate condition of consumption, which killed Keats and played an important part in the premature death of beautiful Vivien Leigh, is now far more likely to come from a cancer of the lung.

Lung cancer is the uncontrolled growth of a gang of cells in the lining of a bronchus, which may or may not cause irritation and coughing early on, but which is likely, quite quickly, to block an airway. The portion of lung beyond the obstruction collapses, and this may mean a disastrous loss of breathing capacity. The situation worsens as the tumor invades farther, causing pain if it involves the pleura or the nerve roots to the chest wall.

Death may follow from suffocation as less and less lung remains serviceable, from infection of the damaged tissue, or from secondary growths affecting vital organs like the brain and liver. These are started by cancer cells from the lung being carried in the bloodstream.

Cancer is the second leading cause of death among people aged forty-five to fifty-four, in advanced economies, and even allowing for changes in the age of the population, it has increased in overall frequency by 10 percent in the last ten years. By far the commonest cancer is cancer of the lung, and in Britain alone it kills thirty thousand people a year: more than fifty a day. Eight times as many of the victims are men as women, and while it can strike down those of forty to fifty, like a coronary, it does so more often at age fifty plus.

Lung cancer, like some others, is one form of reaction to some long-term irritant. There are no prizes for guessing what this irritant is in most cases.

Cancer of the larynx is the little sister of lung cancer. It is not nearly as common, but is on the increase, and again is more likely in men than women, and again is usually caused by cigarette smoke. As you would expect, the voice is affected. The laryx, or voice box, sits at the upper end of the trachea.

Chronic bronchitis with emphysema is another kind of response to an irritant that is inhaled. The mucus-manufacturing glands in the bronchial tubes, which normally provide just enough to keep the airways moist and clean, work overtime in an effort to protect the lungs from the irritant. A vast excess of sticky material coats the bronchial walls and clogs the smaller tubes. Swelling of the lining of the airways adds to the obstruction, and the effect is most obvious when you try to breathe out, normally an effortless affair. Air may be trapped in the tiny, thin-walled air sacs, and they may blow up like miniature balloons and burst; this is the beginning of emphysema.

Sooner or later infecting organisms settle in the mucus-filled, ill-ventilated airways, disorganizing and destroying their structure and that of the surrounding lung tissue. In an attempt to compensate, the surviving parts of the lungs overstretch themselves and the chest remains always expanded, so that less and less extra air can be drawn in with each breath. A winter cough, when there are infections about, and phlegm to bring up are early results of the bronchitic process. Wheezing, and tightness of the chest, especially in the morning, show that the tubes are clobbered by sticky secretions. Breathing becomes progressively more difficult as the wreckage of lung tissue continues.

The deadliest dangers come about because of the inability to get enough air to live, or because of failure of the heart to stand up to its increased work load, i.e., sending blood through the diseased lungs; also, any surgical operation involving an anesthetic may prove too great a strain on the resources of a chronic bronchitic.

Bronchial asthma is a condition which seems at first blink to be very like bronchitis. It is characterized by attacks of wheezing and difficulty in breathing, and often by coughing on exertion. What goes on is a temporary narrowing of the bronchial tubes by a spasm of the muscle in their walls, swelling of the lining, and an increase in sticky mucus secretion. This interferes with the ventilation of the lungs by increasing the resistance to the air flow through the tubes. Breathing out, normally the more passive process, becomes noticeably more difficult. "If I ever get this breath out, I'll never take another one," is how one asthmatic felt as he struggled.

The narrowed tubes are not properly cleared by coughing, so the mucus in them gets half-dried and stickier. When a number of bronchioles are affected, breathing out becomes a conscious and exhausting effort, and may even become impossible. Or the strain on the heart may be more than it can carry. The muscle spasm that causes the essential narrowing of the tubes may be brought on by allergic irritation, infection, or emotion.

Pulmonary infarction may be "no-account" slight or dangerous to the point of death, if a large area of lung is affected. In pulmonary embolism—mentioned *en passant* in the previous chapter—fragments of a clot somewhere else in the body, for instance in a vein or the heart, may be carried in the bloodstream and lodge in the arteries of the lungs, immediately cutting off the blood supply to a section or sections of those organs.

This can happen after a coronary, after an operation, to a woman during pregnancy and after, or to a woman when she is on the pill. Embolism is one type of pulmonary infarction—blocking of the blood supply to part of the lung, as coronary infarction is a similar blocking of the supply to part of the heart muscle. And, like a coronary, pulmonary infarction can also happen through spontaneous clotting (thrombosis) of the blood in a lung artery, which may be atherosclerotic, like any other. Some precipitating causes, such as a fatty meal or anger, as sometimes happens with a coronary thrombosis, may apply.

Lung tissue that has lost its blood supply dies. Several small arteries or one large artery put out of service can cause immediate death, or a very serious situation, complete with shortness of breath, a crushing pain like a coronary, and a feeling of faintness because of lack of oxygenation in the brain. There is a dangerous strain on the right side of the heart and difficulty for the heart as a whole, because of the shortage of oxygen in the blood which supplies it.

These, then, are the main causes that may lead to a disastrous failure of your oxygenating plant. All of them are, to a very large extent, avoidable.

PREDISPOSITION

Far and away the most important predisposing cause of any trouble in the respiratory system is self-inflicted injury by smoking. Colds, coughs, and sinusitis are commoner and last longer if you smoke, because of the paralysis by smoke of the germ-killing cells in the mouth, which are your first line of defense against infection. Because of the paralytic effect of smoke on the cleansing mechanism of the tubes, infection that has breached the defenses of the upper reaches of the respiratory system may the more easily invade the lower, more vital, parts of it and cause laryngitis, bronchitis, and even pneumonia. Such infections may be life-shortening in themselves, or may make another lung condition far more serious. And even a cold in the head can lead to death if it fuddles your wits at some critical moment.

Smoking has a direct, positive association with chronic bronchitis, and although this disease is somewhat more prevalent in polluted urban and industrial milieus, it is on the smokers, in particular, that pollution has its harmful effect. Rats breathing tobacco smoke develop more mucus-making cells in their bronchial tubes—the basis of morning cough.

Smoking has also a statistically causative link with lung cancer—our commonest cancer in an age when cancer is on the increase as a cause of death. From the latest reports it seems that any kind of smoking involves some risk of lung cancer. Animal experiments show that filter tips just don't sieve off the cancer-producing component in the smoke, although they do marginally reduce the bronchitis-producing effect. The death rate from cancer of the lung in heavy cigarette smokers is thirty times that of nonsmokers.

Ex-smokers have an outlook proportionately better, depending on how long they have smoked and how long it has been since they stopped. Currently, our society is obsessed by anxieties about drug addiction, but clearly, nicotine addiction is far more widespread and more lethal, particularly because of its association with atherosclerosis and coronary thrombosis, chronic bronchitis and emphysema, lung cancer, cancer of the larynx, etc. Pulmonary infarction may be indirectly associated with smoking, peptic ulcer is made worse by it, and it slows your reaction time at the wheel.

Polluted air, such as that in a big city, and particularly when a highly irritating smog is formed, as in Los Angeles, Barcelona, and, worst of all, Tokyo, predisposes to breathing troubles.

Industrial dusts, especially those containing abrasives, may cause scarring of the lungs, bronchitis, or lung cancer.

Continuously dry, warm air, as from central heating, or long-wave radiation, as from electric fires, with a lack of stimulating short-wave radiation and cool, moist air, tend to congest the lining of the nose and make it more susceptible to infection.

Pollens, house dust, and other quite ordinary constituents of the air may set off an asthmatic attack.

Heredity: A susceptibility to chronic bronchitis runs in

families, and while cancer in general is not inherited, you run a greater risk of cancer in a particular part, such as the lung, if relatives have had cancers in this area. The allergic tendency that may lead to asthma is certainly something for which you can blame your parents. Your relatives need not have had asthma itself, but any allergic disorder—say hay fever, eczema, nettlerash—indicates the tendency.

Emotions: Upsets, excitements, and anxiety are common precipitants of an asthmatic attack and may forerun a pulmonary thrombosis, while the simple little action that, repeated often enough, can lead to lung cancer, is often set off by anxiety. The Tobacco Research Council's latest Review of Activities reports that the most consistent precondition for smoking is a situation "seen by the individual as presenting or threatening a high degree of stress."

Damp buildings and a damp climate don't help the breathing apparatus to stay healthy.

Any oddity in the shape of the back or chest, or even of the nose, can predispose to infection. Chronic sinusitis and recurrent tonsillitis may provide a reservoir of germs.

Obesity, while not a cause, makes any respiratory embarrassment more embarrassing. It is obvious that you cannot aerate your lungs as efficiently when you are wearing a close-fitting jacket of fat, half an inch thick.

PRE-ACTION

1. Don't smoke. Not a cigar, pipe, cigarillo, or the villain of them all, a cigarette. Don't even sniff snuff. You know *why* not. You know *how* not: see Chapter IV. But just to remind yourself of what tobacco can do, think of King George VI, one of the best monarchs Britain has ever had, and a premature loss to his family and his country. He didn't know the risks he ran by smoking: you do.

2. Don't grow a wrap of fat around your chest, or if you have—*get it off*. Again, Chapter IV.

3. Do get some unpolluted air into your lungs. Going about in a gas mask might help, or having air conditioning indoors, or living out of town—as long as you can stand up to the stresses of commuting. Or you can plan your vacations and your weekends where there is clean air for your lungs. Getting away is good, but driving nose to tail along a highway for the better part of the day does nothing for anyone.

4. If you are an allergic type particularly, avoid dust like the plague. Go in for Scandinavian-style furnishings and (lack of) floor covering, with curtains of glazed materials that don't harbor the dust. Vacuum-clean everywhere, and plan for someone else to dispose of the dust bag. Strip your bed daily—to the mattress—to discourage *Dermatophagoides pteragyssimus*—the minute allergenic mite harbored in most homes, but not in hospitals where the bedding is autoclaved.

5. Go in for lung-expanding exercise, especially if you have ever had an acute chest infection, or if your chest is of an odd shape. Any exercise stretches your lungs, but swimming more than many others.

6. Do breathing exercises, using your ribs and your diaphragm separately. When you find some fresh air, deep-breathe it.

7. Have cool, fresh air in your home, but don't open windows to let in fog or smog. A howling gale through the bedroom, an English upper-class custom, is not essential and not even desirable if you already have bronchitis. Internal ventilation is then best.

8. Avoid infections, such as colds and worse, by insisting on free ventilation, and by stopping short of extreme fatigue in the key months of January and February. You could try lacing your drinks with a load of vitamin C crystal, amounting to a gram a day, as an anticold maneuver, following the unproven theory of Professor Linus Pauling. And if you know you are going to be in close contact with infection for a special period, eat a meal beforehand: it gives your resistance a temporary boost.

9. Take active steps to get rid of infections promptly. Have one day of minimal activity at the beginning of a

cold, and call on the doctor for antibiotics and advice if it shows signs of going down rather than out.

10. Have an area of chronic or recurrent infection dealt with, such as ears, tonsils, sinuses.

11. Have anti-influenza vaccine each winter.

12. Go for a chest X ray every few years, and immediately if you get a yellow warning.

YELLOW WARNING

Be alert to any of these signs:

Clearing your throat more often than usual. May indicate nervousness, or undue production of mucus in the chest, the forerunner perhaps of smoker's cough, with all its implications.

Morning coughing, or coughing when you go to bed, in exhausting and unproductive bouts, may be the flag of chronic bronchitis or asthma; don't put up with *any* cough that continues for weeks.

Spitting: bringing up phlegm is caused by overwork of the bronchial glands and can mean a little cold; it can also indicate big troubles starting up.

Blood streaking the spit usually means nothing much, but check with the doctor to be on the safe side. Pulmonary infarction is just *one* of the important causes of this occurrence.

Pain in the chest: when it is behind the breastbone and accompanied by coughing it usually means a passing infection. Pain in the side, that gets worse when you breathe or cough, means that something is irritating the sensitive covering of the lung, the pleura. This requires a doctor's expert advice.

Shortness of breath, so that you cannot talk and walk as fast as you used to, or breathing that takes a conscious effort or is difficult needs doctoring too. It may be due to some limitation in the lungs—that's how it feels—or to a heart disorder, or equally, to anxiety. There may be an interplay between the psychological and the physical causes.

There are other disorders, of the thyroid gland, for example, or simple anemia, that can cause this difficulty in breathing.

Wheezing should also direct attention to the lungs, and hoarseness that continues for a fortnight needs investigation.

PRE-ACTION AND FIRST AID

If you experience any of the yellow warning signs, go have yourself examined, by your doctor and by X ray. There is a battery of tests that help in sorting out suspected trouble in the breathing system. The larynx can be inspected by an illuminated metal tube or by a mirror at the back of the mouth; the windpipe and large bronchial tubes by an illuminated tube through which samples of tissue may be taken; the pleural covering of the lung through a space between two ribs; special X-ray examination of the bronchial tree may be made after instillation of an opaque oil; microscopic examination of any phlegm for bacteria or for cancer cells is possible; blood and tubercular tests are available . . . all these are methods for calming particular worries or can be signposts for specific treatment.

The most important first aid treatment is the kiss with which we began this chapter: that is anybody's business. But with a system as important as your breathing, your doctor must be involved from the first symptoms or signs in less urgent situations. Generally, however, you can do something to help yourself.

If you have a cough: Encourage it if you are bringing up phlegm, and help the process, if the material is tenacious, by hot drinks or steaming inhalations. Irritating, tiring coughing that produces nothing should be suppressed as far as is possible. Cough drops may help during the day, but a linctus, a syrupy medicine that calms the cough center, is useful at night and in severe cases.

Difficulty in breathing because of air-passage obstruction, as in asthma and bronchitis, may be greatly alleviated by bronchodilator drugs and steroids, but both of these may be dangerous unless you follow your doctor's instructions to the letter.

Chest pain is usually temporarily relieved by a hot-water bottle, an analgesic, and, if necessary, a linctus to reduce coughing.

Fever with cough should be treated with respect. Get to bed and get medical help. Infections in this vital system can still be deadly if you don't get treatment in time, or if you make physical demands when your body is fighting this infection. Most of the sudden deaths among young soldiers in training occur when a man makes an effort while he has what seems a mild respiratory infection.

THE CRUNCH

BARRY GOODFELLOW: LUNG CANCER

"I haven't a hope in Hell," wrote journalist Mark Waters four days before his death: he had lung cancer like Cannon, the British trades union leader, who died in 1971, and in whose name a cancer-research fund has been set up.

Barry Goodfellow had lung cancer, too. He was an architect whose special talent lay in domestic design, and his own riverside home was one of the most beautiful I have ever seen. Barry smoked on the job, and as he loved his work that meant often. His wife and two pretty daughters made spasmodic efforts to wean him away from his cigarettes, but he was such a good-natured charmer that none of them could bring herself to be stern and unpleasant enough. And there were plenty of arguments the other way; particularly the one that goes that while a large proportion of smokers develop lung cancer, the majority do not. Besides, Barry himself, whose hobby was an outdoor one of fooling around with boats, seemed obviously fit.

When he had a bout of influenza that went to his chest following a busy spell supervising some construction work during damp weather, no one thought it particularly significant. He picked up rather slowly, and his doctor arranged a chest X ray without any real expectation of finding anything wrong. The balloon went up.

A dense, fairly well circumscribed opacity shadowed the outer part of his right lung field. This was not the sort of case where an examination of the bronchial tube from above could be applied. It was too near the outside of the lung. But the chest consultant who was called in had little doubt of the diagnosis. He in turn discussed the matter with a thoracic surgeon. Barry's cancer, for so it proved to be, was fortunately localized in one lobe of one lung. He was otherwise fit and the rest of his breathing system was in good condition, able to carry on the function of oxygenation adequately without the diseased portion. At fifty-two he was comparatively young.

Barry was among the 20 percent of lung-cancer patients considered operable. Resection of the affected lobe was carried out. This was back in 1967, so it seems that Barry has a fair chance of becoming one of the 30 percent who survive the operation after five years, and who can count themselves cured.

Barry can't work or play as hard as he used to, and it's a worry every time he catches a cold, but at least his family, his friends, and his colleagues are grateful to have alive a particularly pleasant and courageous companion. His case is in some ways reminiscent of the British actor Jack Hawkins. His cancer, also contributed to by the cigarette habit, got him in the most devastating area for an actor—the larynx, or voice organ—as was the case with the deep-voiced comedian-singer Jetsam. The latter died. Frederick III of Germany was another well-known figure who smoked, had a laryngeal cancer, and died.

Jack Hawkins underwent the delicate modern operation of laryngectomy, removal of the larynx, and immediately went back to work, at first in nonspeaking parts, and later, having learned to speak from his stomach, in ordinary film parts. His successful recovery is an inspiration and encouragement to anyone who fears he has a cancer from smoking and would hesitate to be operated on.

ELLIS MITCHELL: BRONCHIAL ASTHMA

Looking back he could see that the tendency had been there years before, when he was a teen-ager during World War II. There had been a gas-mask drill, and he found that while everyone else was unaffected, he felt suffocated, and he struggled to breathe even when he had torn the thing off.

However, he went through his National Service—actually after the war—without any trouble, took some accountancy exams while he was still in the RAF, and finally settled down to civilian life in the head office of a chain-store firm. Ellis was a conscientious, orderly worker and it upset him deeply when his immediate boss unfairly gave him a dressing down for some supposed error, in front of an office full of juniors. Ellis did not defend himself, but suppressed his resentment—and developed asthma.

At the time, it seemed that his bouts of breathlessness had come out of the blue. He noticed that breathing out was very slow at these times, and he began to cough, wheeze, and pant on any physical exertion. Of course, his doctor prescribed for him a battery of different drugs: bronchodilators, dicromoglycate, steroids, and emergency medicines for severe attacks. He was given antibiotics promptly when infection complicated the scene. Success was mediocre.

To cut down the possibility of allergenic irritation, Ellis and his wife reorganized their home according to the booklet given by their doctor to anyone with respiratory system allergy. It read like this:

PRECAUTIONS TO BE TAKEN BY THOSE WITH ALLERGY AFFECTING THE NOSE OR CHEST

The commonest causes of respiratory allergy are pollens, molds, feathers, house dust, and the house-dust mite.

Concentrate on making your bedroom as dust-free as possible, since it is the most important room for you: you spend longer in this room than in any other in the twenty-four hours. If you are a hay-fever sufferer or otherwise sensitive to pollens, you must not have any flowers in your room, you should avoid grassy fields and spend your summer vacation by the sea instead.

The bedroom should be as bare as possible, like a cell. Remove all ornaments, pictures, and other dust-catchers. Have light chintz or plastic curtains, oiled linoleum on the floor, or washable plastic, no thick carpets, but perhaps a washable cotton rug.

Furniture should be plain—wooden or metal—sponged weekly. No cloth-covered box springs. Wash woodwork, floor, radiators. Clean picture moldings, if any, with an oiled or damp cloth, and don't allow bedsprings or the back of the wardrobe or chest of drawers to harbor dust. Fitted, built-in furniture is best.

Blankets should be made of Acrilan or cotton. Sew on an extra half length of sheet to your top sheet, or buy very large ones which can be turned over the bed to cover the blankets.

Pillows, bolsters, eiderdown, or mattress should not contain feathers. Use foam rubber pillows, etc., or put pillows in plastic bags, sealed with Scotch tape, until you change them.

Mattress: You may well be allergic to the house-dust mite which lives on mattresses and eats sloughed-off scales of human skin. These mites are best removed by vacuum-cleaning the mattress weekly and by airing the mattress outdoors when it is sunny. Someone else, preferably, should do this.

Cleaning: Use a vacuum cleaner, preferably the cylinder type, to clean the house, and have someone else remove the disposable bag, out of doors if possible. Wear a paper surgical mask if you must do any dusting or vacuuming yourself.

Shaving: Do not use an electric razor because the fine hairs may be breathed in.

Dandruff—your own or your wife/husband's. Get rid of this by energetic treatment with medicated shampoos.

Go on vacation while the house is being redecorated. Dry rot, damp wallpaper, and damp furniture may bring on symptoms.

For some time it seemed that these precautions were making a real difference: then Ellis had a prolonged asthmatic attack and nearly died from it. This happened shortly before he was to have an interview with the superior he disliked; this gave his doctor a clue. Ellis's asthma has improved greatly since he has been helped to develop healthier ways of expressing his bitter antiboss feelings, and he has changed his job. His trend toward danger has gone into reverse; his attacks are far less frequent, and less severe. This is just one asthmatic's experience. For others, particular attention to the allergic or infectious aspects might be more helpful. But for *any* asthmatic, taking trouble can repay with a years-long dividend. Ellis is now forty-nine.

MAISIE BRADBERRY: CHRONIC BRONCHITIS

In 1969 there were thirty thousand deaths from chronic bronchitis in the United Kingdom. Maisie might have been one of the departed. She was a plump, easygoing widow of fifty who helped out, on a short-term, high-fee basis, families in which the mother was ill or had just given birth. She could turn her hand to anything, from giving a baby his bottle to whipping up a cake—with a faint flavor of ashes from the cigarettes she perpetually smoked.

People put up with her habit of simultaneously smoking and cooking because she was so responsible, and such a comfortable person to have around. Her winter cough, at first slight, became increasingly troublesome with each successive winter from about 1964 on, and every time she had a cold she developed an attack of acute bronchitis. In due course, she became continuously wheezy, and her chest felt uncomfortably tight first thing in the morning before the sticky mucus in her bronchial tubes had been cleared by hot tea and hard coughing. As her breathing reserves were encroached upon more and more she began to be noticeably breathless, and what had been no effort was now exhausting.

The course which led Maisie away from the slippery slope to death included:

1. Stopping smoking.
2. Moving from the city's polluted atmosphere to a less well paid job in purer air. It was sunnier, too.
3. Taking off thirty pounds.
4. Taking antibiotic treatment promptly for every respiratory infection, however slight, since each such episode can do further and permanent damage to the lungs. Her doctor gave her a supply of tablets to have always at hand, and the dosage he recommended was a generous one.
5. Sleeping always in a warm bedroom, with ventilation coming through an open door rather than through the window.
6. Taking a cough suppressant at night, when her cough was tickling and unproductive, to save herself from tiring effort and the disturbance of her sleep.
7. Taking a hot drink first thing in the morning.

Now, at fifty-six, five years older and five years fitter, it looks as though Maisie has the main dangers of her chest condition under control. She certainly looks—and sounds—years younger.

ANDY STAMP: PULMONARY INFARCTION

Andy had his trouble when he was forty-six: a sudden pain in his chest that made him think he had a coronary, breathlessness that was better when he lay flat, and a feeling of faintness. He was treated in the hospital with an anticoagulant drip into his bloodstream to discourage any further clotting, and he came out with anticoagulant tablets to take for a few months.

In this particular disaster there is usually no time to do anything to save life if the blood supply to a large area of lung is cut off at a single blow. Andy came through the first attack. But there is a 20 to 30 percent likelihood of recurrence of pulmonary infarction, and so it has been important for him to reverse the process of atherosclerosis which had led him to the brink of tragedy. After the anticoagulants had tided him over the short-term dangers he was on his own, depending on a changed diet and living habits to keep himself out of the woods. Less food, less fat—unless polyunsaturated—less stress, more exercise, and additional breathing exercises as a tonic to his lungs after the insult to them, made up the basic style of his new life.

It seems that the style was right, since no further attack has troubled Andy, despite the busy and demanding life he leads as a TV personality.

7

Kidneys and Bladder

Kidney failure kills at any age, from childhood on, and accounts for thousands of premature deaths, despite modern advances and the dramatic successes of dialysis and transplant.

Physically, the kidneys are just the shape they always are in pictures, unlike the formal hearts you see on a St. Valentine's Day card, which bear no resemblance to the actual human organ. Each kidney is about four and a half inches long, two and a half inches wide, and one and one half inches deep, and weighs about five ounces. The kidneys are not situated in the loins, but are higher up, and safer, just in front of the root of the twelfth rib, snug to the spine. Two tubes, the ureters, run down from them to the bladder, or urine tank, and this has a single piped outflow.

Basically, the kidney is a black box for keeping correct the mineral balance of your body, whether you down sixteen beers an evening or play six sets of tennis and lose fluid in your sweat. Your kidneys also eliminate unwanted and potentially dangerous wastes from the body, so long as these are soluble in water. Foreign substances that get into the bloodstream, including drugs taken when you are ill, are picked out and discarded by the kidneys. The exact composition of the body fluids is vital to your existence, and death from kidney failure is due to derangements in this composition. This is seen by the striking efficacy of dialysis, or use of the artificial kidney machine. An artificial kidney is basically a sheet of cellophane through which the blood is filtered. The natural kidney is a filtering apparatus too, but a thousand times more complex, involving about 1,250,000 filtration units, each served by selector tubes which take back into the circulation the substances the body wants after all.

The process is like getting your desk tidy by sweeping everything off it and then putting back only the things you actually need; this is what your kidneys do to your blood. For instance, sugar and water are both withdrawn from the blood as it circulates through the kidney filters, but are grabbed back again when it reaches the tubules. You may have noticed that in cold weather you pass more and paler urine: the tubules don't function as well when it is chilly, and they take back less water.

Waste products come largely from the combustion of food on which the body runs. Fats and carbohydrates break down into water, and the gas carbon dioxide is easily discharged through the lungs in your breath. But protein presents more of a problem. Fish solve it by converting it into ammonia and releasing this into the sea. We turn protein into a soluble compound called *urea* and excrete it in the urine. This substance is poisonous if it accumulates in the body, and if you are not eating much protein your kidneys don't have to produce as much urine in order to carry it away.

It is a measure of the importance of the kidneys that they receive a quarter of the total output of blood from the heart: thirteen hundred milliliters pass through each minute. Where the complexity of the kidneys pays off, as compared with a simpler filter system, is in their capacity to control their activity to suit the body's moment-to-moment requirements. Their double countercurrent mechanism can dispose of extra fluid if you drink deep, or conserve your water supply if you are in the Sahara, have diarrhea, or run a fever. The average daily output of the kidneys is eight hundred to thirteen hundred milliliters, but this can vary with the circumstances. Whatever the volume, the amount of solid matter excreted remains constant at about two ounces a day.

Multiple feedback makes the kidney system highly sensitive to its own progress, and its ability to evaluate constantly the volume and exact chemical constitution of the blood enables it to control which functions to perform, and how intensively to pursue a particular course. Your kidneys' remarkable power of keeping your internal chemistry steady is what enables you to survive a trip to equatorial Africa or the Arctic, or a limited period without food or water. Kidney function controls our thirst. In health, this makes us drink at least enough to carry off the urea in the blood, and if the kidney fails and urea accumulates, one of the most distressing symptoms is a raging thirst.

One of the most important minerals in the blood is sodium chloride—common salt—in fact, it gives the blood its salty taste. The output of salt from the body is managed by the kidneys. If you lose a lot of blood, say in an accident, there is a sharp reduction in the amount of salt and water that your kidneys release: you may need it all to make up the loss. If you are standing still and upright your body retains more salt and water, and in such circumstances your ankles may swell with the fluid. But when you lie down your kidneys get rid of more salt, and not so much fluid is kept in the body.

Diuretics are substances which increase the flow of urine. You probably have taken one today—as tea, coffee, or cocoa. There are also medicinal diuretics, including the newest, like frusemide, which act by blocking the reabsorption of salt and water already selected out. These drugs are useful in ridding the body of excess fluid.

A day in the life of your kidneys is varied and complex, and one of their unexpected functions is the production of a hormone called renin. Through a chain of reactions this leads to the manufacture of another chemical that keeps the blood pressure down. Damage or disease of the kidneys is often accompanied by a rise in the blood pressure.

HOW THEY CAN GO WRONG

Your kidneys, sensitive, delicate, complicated, are built to operate at a certain pressure of the blood. If your blood pressure falls drastically, as it may with blood loss or shock, your kidneys can't work and you may die. This is an emergency situation, and one reason why, when I asked a well-known surgeon what he would recommend for a first-aid kit, he suggested a tracheotomy tube and a drip and nothing else—the former to provide an air passage, and the latter a method of getting fluid into the circulation and raising the blood pressure. For the rest of us, with neither a drip nor the expertise to use it, the best treatment for someone in shock is to provide adequate warmth by covering him with a blanket (no hot-water bottles), and giving him a bland, nonalcoholic drink, especially if there has been a loss of fluid from bleeding or from an extensive burn. This may save kidney function, and life.

Much more likely than a disaster that puts your blood pressure too low for your kidneys' health is the condition of high blood pressure, either sporadic or constant. Any rise in the blood pressure inevitably damages your kidneys. The kidney attempts to protect itself through its autoregulation mechanism: clamping down its arteries and reducing the blood flow through them. Long-standing high blood pressure gradually destroys the kidneys: the vital working units shrink and scar up, and the whole kidney becomes smaller and is no longer functional.

The reduced blood flow through the kidneys when their arteries tighten up in response to raised blood pressure means that they make less renin, and this in turn means that the blood pressure becomes higher. A vicious circle of mounting blood pressure and increasing kidney damage is set up. The high blood pressure may be the greater danger because it involves the risk of stroke, hypertensive heart failure, or coronary attack, although damage to the kidneys may turn out to be fatal as well. This is most probable if there has been kidney disease in the past.

Acute nephritis is a serious infection of the kidney. Anyone can get it and it is likely to come on about three weeks after a streptococcal infection of the throat or some other part of the breathing system. This may have been so mild you took no account of it. A pale, puffy face, blood in the urine, and a general feeling of being ill, with loss of appetite, fever, and headache, usher the condition in. The doctor will clinch the diagnosis by finding the raised blood pressure, and by examination of the urine. This illness should be taken seriously. Ninety percent of children, but only 50 percent of adults, recover completely in a week or two. The unlucky ones progress to:

Chronic nephritis: This is a slowly developing death of the kidneys, usually associated with raised blood pressure. It is not always preceded by acute nephritis. The composition of the body fluids goes haywire if the kidney fails in its functions, and every part of the body feels the effects. The owner feels tired, thirsty, and weak, and finds he has to pass more water than usual, at night as well as during the day.

Chronic nephritis is a deadly disease for which heroic treatments such as transplants and dialysis have been introduced. Even without these, however, there is hope, as we shall see.

Acute pyelonephritis: This is an acute inflammation of the collecting funnel (pelvis) of the kidney, as opposed to the main functional part, that is affected in acute nephritis. It usually crops up because of some obstruction to the outflow of urine, lower down. For instance, it is relatively common at about the fifth month of pregnancy, or may arise if a man's prostate gland becomes enlarged in middle age, or it may come about because of stones or tumors in the bladder.

Women are more susceptible than men to this trouble

because of their shorter urine tube, allowing infection to ascend more easily. Pyelonephritis comes on suddenly with pain in one or both loins, streaking around to the front of the abdomen, and a high fever. Sometimes there is fever but no pain. The illness usually clears up rapidly. leaving no trace, but treated inadequately it can slip into a chronic condition, the cause of vague bad health for years, and ultimately leading, perhaps, to chronic nephritis. It is not to be taken too lightly.

Cystitis: A common infection of the bladder. You don't feel ill in general, but you have to pass water frequently and it is painful. Often you have an intense desire to pass more urine, but the bladder is empty—a condition aptly called *strangury.* Cystitis, like a cold in the head, isn't a killing disease, but it may be an indication of more serious disease either of the kidney or at the base of the bladder. Obstruction to the outflow of urine means stagnation, and this foreshadows not only cystitis but also bladder cancer, so it is important to pinpoint and deal with it.

Cystitis that lingers on or recurs involves a constant risk of infection creeping up the urine tubes and reaching the kidneys, causing damage to these vital organs; so not even cystitis can safely be neglected.

Cancer of the bladder: This is the commonest cancer of the urinary system and it is on the increase. Ninety-four percent of victims of this form of cancer have smoked more than ten cigarettes a day for more than ten years: smoking increases the excretion of certain cancer-stimulating bodily waste products. Some industrial fumes may act in the same way, and certain aromatic amines have a proven relationship to bladder cancer. If you have any reason to come in contact with 2-naphthalene and 4-aminobiphenyl, for instance, be wary.

Some bladder tumors are harmless in themselves but may develop malignancy and become killers unless treated promptly. Anything that impedes the outflow of urine makes cancer likelier because the cancer-producing substances become concentrated while they wait in the bladder. Enlargement of the prostate gland is one cause of a slow-emptying bladder.

Enlargement of the prostate gland: This can be harmless or cancerous. Either way, it tends to crop up at fifty plus. Obstruction to the outflow of urine is the main result of enlargement of this sex gland at the base of the bladder. This can cause stagnation, which, as in the village pond, is unhealthy, leading to infection, stone formation, or cancer. Any back pressure on the kidneys can deter their efficient functioning, and even cause kidney failure.

Naturally, if your prostate becomes oversize either malignantly, or, as is far more likely, benignly, you have water problems. Having to get up in the night is one of the first symptoms. A poor stream, and difficulty in starting (although you are desperate to get there) and stopping, are others. Benign prostatic enlargement happens only to man and his domestic dog. It can lead to your death indirectly if you don't take steps. Its bad brother, cancer of the prostate, can do so directly if not treated, but treatment for this cancer—by hormones—is most effective.

PRE-ACTION

To keep your kidneys and urinary system serving you safely, you need do only six things:

1. Keep them primed with fluids, particularly when you have lost or are losing fluid: urgently in burns or blood loss, but also in feverishness, vomiting, and diarrhea, and with copious sweating.

2. Avoid the indirect poisoning of tobacco smoke and the industrial substances mentioned above.

3. If you are taking a medicine that could harm your kidneys, then at least drink plenty of fluids while you are on it. Such medicines include various antibiotics of which the only commonly used one is tetracycline (penicillin and erythromycin are in the clear); bismuth salts; phenacetin (used still in some analgesic tablets); gold salts; and sulfa drugs. Antihistamines and sedatives may cause retention

of urine and hence kidney damage. However, most people are not sensitive to any of these medicines.

4. Take notice of any symptoms which could be connected with kidney or urinary trouble; act immediately, and persevere with any treatment prescribed.

5. Regular checks of the urine during pregnancy, especially from the fourth month onward, are recommended.

6. Blood pressure checks should be run from time to time.

YELLOW WARNING

Troubles in the kidneys often don't show up immediately in those glands, but there are plenty of pointers:

1. Frequency of passing water, without discomfort (commonest cause is anxiety).

2. Having to rise at night to pass water.

3. Blood in the water: may be red, but more likely the urine merely looks smoky. Red or dark urine urgently needs investigating, but the commonest causes are not serious diseases but black currants, blackberries, beetroot, candies, or medicines dyed red.

4. Unpleasant-smelling urine: may be infection, may be asparagus.

5. Swelling of the face, headaches, lassitude: any of these calls for a trip to the doctor to check for kidney disease.

6. Pain or discomfort on passing water, usually frequently.

7. Pain in the loins, perhaps extending to the front.

8. Urgency to pass water—you can't wait. The doctor may find other interesting signs of trouble, such as high blood pressure or sugar or protein in the urine.

Signs of the kidney in desperate need of help: Flatulent dyspepsia; loss of weight; thirst; dry, dirty tongue; lassitude and inability to concentrate; nervousness and irritability —continuing on, and not the occasional result of a night out.

THE CRUNCH

The minor crunches, those circumstances that could lead on to a major disaster, should be treated, like your rich aunt, with respect. With any *infection* of the urinary tract, be meticulous in following treatment and in having follow-up checks later. Sometimes you need to be on suppressive therapy for months or years.

With any *obstruction* to outflow get it corrected promptly, however inconvenient.

With any *blood* in the urine don't waste time. Whatever the trouble it can be dealt with a lot more effectively if caught early.

Chronic nephritis: If it comes to this diagnosis, that is the serious crunch. You must consider your kidney as a delicate invalid. Your doctor will take steps to reduce your blood pressure, probably with tablets. You can help by keeping your temper in the short run and your anxieties down in the long. Your doctor will also advise you on diet, according to how much protein he thinks your kidney can cope with. An ordinary British-American diet allows eighty to one hundred grams of protein daily. Cutting this to forty or sixty grams takes an appreciable load off your kidneys. (Around twenty grams daily is the minimum.)

A diet such as this would help a mild to moderate case of kidney failure:

BREAKFAST
Cornflakes and fruit, with milk from allowance;[1] 1 egg,
2 pieces of bacon, or *small* helping of fish;
1½ thin slices of toast, marmalade;
Butter and milk from allowance;
Tea or coffee with milk from allowance, and sugar.

MIDMORNING
Tea or coffee with milk from allowance, sugar, or fruit
juice with glucose. Plain cracker.

---

[1] *Allowance for day:* 1 pint milk; 2 ounces butter.

LUNCH
Small helping of meat, poultry, game, fish;
Helping of vegetables; helping of potatoes;
Milk pudding with milk from allowance;
Fruit, fresh, stewed, or tinned.

MIDAFTERNOON
1 thin sandwich of cucumber, tomato, date, banana, or
    jam;
Butter and milk from allowance;
Tea.

DINNER
1 egg, poached, boiled, scrambled; or part of tomato,
    asparagus, or spinach omelet; or *small* helping of
    macaroni and cheese, or fish cake;
Vegetables if desired;
Milk pudding with milk from allowance, or fruit;
1½ thin slices of bread, jam, jelly, honey;
Butter and milk from allowance;
Coffee.

No salt to be added at table and the minimum to be
used in cooking if blood pressure is raised or if there is
any swelling of the ankles or face.

If there is a tendency to accumulation of fluid in the
tissues then it is usually wise to restrict salt intake. Curries
are spicy but not salty, incidentally, and very suitable.

It takes resolve to keep to a restricted diet, but the
prize may be survival. Although kidney transplants and
renal dialysis—the so-called artificial kidney—can be life-
saving *in extremis,* in milder cases it is sufficient to pamper
the kidneys dietetically for a long stretch. Even in severe
cases, persistence with the right diet can lead to some
recovery of kidney function and ultimately a return to a
near-normal diet.

*If you have a kidney disorder, do get advice from one
of the top ten renal experts in your country.*

IRWIN SCHULTZ: ACUTE GLOMERULONEPHRITIS

Irwin was a stationery salesman for a firm that was up and coming but hadn't quite got there. Consequently, he could afford to miss no opportunities. If he had a sore throat he didn't have time to bother about it. As far as he was concerned it all came out of the blue: he woke up one fine morning to feel his face oddly fat and stiff and he felt awful: nauseated, headachy, feverish. When he went to the bathroom his urine looked sinisterly smoky. On his way back, he looked in the mirror and saw a pasty, puffy face, not improved by its morning bristle.

This was serious. He staggered back into bed clutching the phone and rang his girl friend to tell her he was dying and that she had better come quick. She did.

In fact he was in no immediate danger, although he was in considerable discomfort; there was, however, a fair long-term risk that this acute kidney infection would lead on to chronic nephritis and kidney failure later on. Marcia steered him away from this precipice by making it possible for him to follow his doctor's advice and keeping him to it: rest and warmth and no drafts; bed rest for four weeks—by which time his urine had returned to normal and the swelling had subsided; dietary regulation: restricted drinking of all kinds; food as he fancied so long as he didn't fancy protein; bread, cereals, biscuits, butter and jam, fruit and vegetables were all allowed; no added salt. Antibiotics over a five-day period were prescribed.

After he was recovered he had removed an elderly molar which an X ray showed as a probable reservoir of infection. And Irwin did marry the girl, which he might have done sooner. He should have no further trouble.

BRETT PARSONS:
CHRONIC GLOMERULONEPHRITIS

This man was vicar of a parish in a part of London noted for its violence and vandalism. It was a demanding job, but Brett had the crusading spirit, a wife who was a help and support, and four delightful children. At first he seemed equal to anything, then gradually he found himself always tired and exhausted at the slightest physical effort, and he was only forty-four.

Brett was a friend of mine, and when I saw him in 1969 he was living on intermittent dialysis, an unpalatable twenty-five-gram protein diet, and despair. His kidneys were giving out. He was being moved from his busy parish to a tiny country village, suitable for an invalid. We lost touch.

In spring 1971, I chanced to be driving in that part of the country, and I thought I would visit Brett—or his widow, I didn't know which I should find. I was amazed and delighted to discover that Brett had just returned from a grueling tour of the Holy Land and was looking perfectly normal, and had returned to nearly normal eating habits. His is a case of recovery by dietary and medical means alone. His children will have a father after all, and his wife will be a happy, struggling parson's wife, rather than a sad, struggling widow.

ANTHEA IDDINGS: BLADDER CANCER

Anthea was the manageress of a tobacconist's shop for thirty years, as well as working as a housewife and mother of two. Of course she smoked: it was one of the perquisites of the job. She had had one or two attacks of cystitis, including one when she was expecting Charlie, her second son. Both attacks had cleared up fairly quickly. It was after a party with some of her husband's friends that she first noticed blood in her urine: it came at the end of her passing water. She felt perfectly well, and the next time it didn't happen, so she did nothing. Then the blood showed up again, and she began to worry and lie awake. After two or three nights of this her husband was alerted to her worries.

With blood in the urine every day's delay means added danger. The cause may be an innocent tumor: innocent at present. Even an early cancer is much easier to remove than one that has developed. The urological surgeon who investigated Anthea found a single, fairly superficial tumor and decided on transurethral electroresection: that is, via the urine tube. There is a 70 percent chance of cure at this stage, and for Anthea three years have already gone by uneventfully since her operation. The outlook for her is good, but had she waited, her chances with the resection treatment would have been only 30 percent for a five-year survival. A drug treatment is now beginning to be used for this kind of cancer, but the tumor must be attended to early with this as well as with resection surgery.

8

Diabetes and
Its Complications

It must have been pretty plushy in ancient Egypt. *Diabetes mellitus* was described there some 3500 years ago in the Ebers Papyrus, and we know that diabetes is a disease of prosperity. We think that it affects more than 1 percent of today's population in the affluent West, but not all the cases are detected. The most important factor leading to the prevalence of diabetes is the opportunity to eat too much, especially of sugars and starches. When food was scarce in Europe during World War II, there were fewer cases of diabetes. It is less common among the natives in struggling India than among those who have settled in South Africa. (In Durban, in particular, the people are noted for the large amounts of sugar they consume.)

The death rate from diabetes is going up. In the United States 106 people died from it in 1969 for every 100 who died in 1964–68.

WHAT IS DIABETES?

The pancreas is a soft, pinkish gland, tucked away by the first bend of the intestine. It produces an important digestive juice, and an even more important compound called *insulin*. This is released into the bloodstream and has an effect throughout the body, concerned as it is with the latter's fuel consumption.

In the ordinary course of events, food is taken into the body, processed, and then burned in order to power its activities—from running to thinking. The food is of three types: carbohydrates (sugars and starches); proteins (meats, fish, eggs, cheese); and fats. Carbohydrates are the main fuel, however, and circulate in the blood, ready for use, as sugar. The function of insulin is to enable the tissues to take in immediately the glucose they require for slow combustion; to assist in the formation of glycogen, which is a compact way of storing carbohydrate for future use; and to help in the conversion of carbohydrate into fat, the long-term deposit of energy. The circulating glucose is like the money in your pocket, the glycogen like the cash in your checking account, and the fat your savings account.

In diabetes, the pancreas does not, for one reason or another, produce enough insulin. The result is that the diabetic has the terrible handicap of being unable to use sugar and starches properly, and these are the body's main fuel in diets anywhere in the world. The sugar that cannot be burned up properly accumulates in the blood, overflows through the kidney, and is poured out as waste in the urine. The excess, unusable sugar poisons the victim, and the shortage of fuel makes him feel weak. Because the blood is so full of sugar the diabetic feels thirsty—you know how thirsty you feel if you have been guzzling chocolates. Because there is so much sugar, he has to pass a lot of urine to get rid of some of it.

Since a severe diabetic cannot use the sugars and starches in his diet efficiently, he may have to burn fats and proteins excessively for vital fuel. The trouble with this is it may produce certain poisonous acids in the body, called ketone bodies. The effect of these is to cause vomiting, sleepiness, coma, and, finally, death, unless he is treated. If it were not for this, it would be quite simple to deal with diabetes merely by cutting down on the carbohydrate in the diet and replacing it with protein and fat. As it is, the whole diet of a diabetic must be tailored to suit him.

When the pancreas is working normally it has a feedback system which enables it to provide the output of insulin that is needed to deal with the exact amount of carbohydrate eaten. In a mild case of diabetes it may be able to produce enough to deal with small amounts of carbohydrate; in a slightly more severe case a tablet which may stimulate the pancreas to its best efforts can be enough to control the situation; but in severe cases the body urgently needs a supply of insulin imported from outside.

DIABETES CAN KILL

It can do it directly if there is no treatment, or if the treatment is careless, through diabetic coma. It also fosters complications which are dangerous.

Atherosclerosis affects everybody to some extent, but diabetics are particularly prone to it because of the larger than normal amounts of fat in their blood. Atherosclerosis consists of deposits of fat in the artery walls, and it is the parent of coronary attacks and strokes. In diabetics it also commonly affects the arteries to the limbs, and may even lead to gangrene.

Infections are common in diabetics because the sugar richness fosters bacterial growth. Carbuncles, tuberculosis of the lungs, and urinary infections are examples. Any of these can have serious consequences.

Kidney disease is another dangerous complication of diabetes, and characteristic of it, but not immediately dangerous, are eye disorders and itching of the skin.

PREDISPOSING CONDITIONS

Diabetes comes in two "styles": early-onset and maturity-onset types. The early type comes on in childhood or adolescence as a rule and affects males more than females. It is usually severe, requiring insulin, and has a definite genetic link.

The maturity-onset type is far commoner, appears at forty plus and affects mainly women. It is milder, and does not run in families, so far as can be discovered.

Although there are many fat people who are not diabetic, most middle-aged diabetics are overweight. They are often those with an especially sweet tooth, and it seems reasonable to suppose that they have put too great a strain on insulin production, so that it has failed. Various conditions, though not strictly causative, may bring diabetes out into the open for the first time. An infection, for instance, throws an extra strain on the insulin-producing cells, and may reveal a latent case. Stress, as from a fearful car crash, may also appear to precipitate diabetes, as may a surgical operation, or a steroid treatment for some other disorder.

Hormone disturbances, for instance those of pregnancy, or an overactive thyroid gland, may bring on diabetes. So may liver disease, and certain drugs. Inflammation of the pancreas or other damage to it are rare causes.

AVOIDING DIABETES

Avoid having the wrong parents. Avoid being a woman. Avoid being married, if a woman—or unmarried, if a man. Avoid motherhood. Avoid middle age . . .

Apart from these hints from the dustbin of statistics, the only truly avoidable factor seems to be overweight; it's back to the old line of eating a good deal less and exercising a good deal more. In particular, carbohydrates should be taken in moderation since it is too much of these that is likely to overtax the pancreas. A list of foods very rich in carbohydrates is at the end of this chapter. Too much fat in the diet, on the other hand, may accelerate the development of atherosclerosis, a major complication in diabetes itself. So it looks like lean meat and a lettuce leaf pretty often is the thing.

Screening is an excellent way to pick up incipient diabetes at an early stage, before it has done any harm. Prompt correction of the tendency avoids, if not the disease, at least its dangers. Screening, if you need reminding, is a medical examination including a battery of special tests, which is done to find out about hidden disorders and weak points in a person's health before he has noticed any definite symptoms. A good fortieth-birthday present for your body.

THE CRUNCH

Suppose you have had some of these nine symptoms:

1. Excessive quantities of urine
2. Unusual thirst
3. Loss of weight
4. Hunger
5. Weakness
6. Fatigue
7. Itching
8. Trouble with your sight
9. Boils and skin infections.

Just two or three of these symptoms should be enough to send you to your doctor for a checkup. It will include urine tests for sugar and ketones, blood-sugar tests, and tolerance curves. These will lead to the verdict. If it *is* diabetes you are in for a lifetime of treatment, but it isn't a death warrant—not even a slow-acting one if you follow the rules. Treatment consists of:

1. Diet alone, or
2. Diet and tablets, or
3. Diet and insulin injections.

Get the message? It is diet that counts, whatever else, and it must be designed to fit *you*—middle years and plump; middle years and average weight; or young and active. The proportion of food from each category— carbohydrate, protein, and fat—must be balanced to suit your type and activity. Commonly, it works out 40 percent carbohydrate; 15 percent protein; and 45 percent fat.

Vitamins: A diabetic diet with its emphasis on fruit, vegetables, and high-protein and fat-content foods is likely to supply generously all the vitamins required. The possible exception is the B group, and some diabetics need supplements of these.

The mildest of diabetics may not need to have a formal diet at all, but may merely have to cut out the highly concentrated carbohydrate foods. Many others merely need to discover a diet that suits them and that keeps sugar out of their urine, and then to stick to it. Tablets—the originals were tolbutamide and chlorpropamide—help mild, middle-aged cases mainly, in which diet alone nearly clears the sugar from the urine; they do *not* help severe cases and may even make matters worse by acting to stimulate the failing pancreas, but no one is sure about this.

The life-saving mainstay of treatment in diabetes is insulin, a replacement for the natural product, and it is only effective through injection. Most diabetics soon learn the skill of self-injection so that they think no more of it than of brushing their teeth.

HOW NOT TO DIE YOUNG WITH DIABETES

Any diabetic who wants to live well and long must discipline himself and abide by certain rules. Doing this will enable him to do more of what he likes as well as make him feel fitter.

1. Regularity in living matters more to the diabetic than to most.
2. Moderation in all things, plenty of rest, and an "off" switch as far as worry goes. Stress of any sort is bad for the diabetic.
3. Mild exercise: certainly good. Vigorous exercise needs your doctor's O.K.
4. Keeping the bowels regular: the fruit and vegetables should do this.
5. Avoid colds, sore throats, and flu. Infections make diabetes worse.
6. Scrupulous cleanliness of the skin, and especially the feet. Skin infections are common and harmful in diabetes. Use a qualified chiropodist for any foot disorders.
7. Check to see that any medicines used don't contain undue amounts of sugar—for instance, cough syrup. (Sugar-coated pills contain only negligible amounts.)
8. Keep to the prescribed diet, and don't take liberties. Weigh the foods now and again to check your rough estimate of portions.
9. Carry out urine tests yourself, twice a week. If they are bad, get medical advice.
10. If you are on insulin, look after your syringe hygienically; be meticulous about the timing of your injections, and don't use the same area of skin twice running. Check the expiration date on your insulin bottle.
11. Learn how to adjust your insulin to unusual amounts of exercise, or when your diet has been put awry, for instance by Yom Kippur, or by any difficulty in getting the correct foods.

EMERGENCY SITUATIONS

You and your family must know how to cope with these:

Hypoglycemia is caused by too much insulin for the available sugar. This can occur if an overdose of insulin is taken accidentally or the normal amount of carbohydrate is not eaten, or extra exercise has used it up; or if your diabetes is naturally improving, as happens in some cases. The signs are a weak, slack, shaky, dizzy, nervous feeling; hot or cold sweat; maybe hunger; maybe palpitation; tingling of lips or hands. Any of these sensations calls for immediate action: take sugar—the two lumps that should always be in your pocket—with water, and rest for fifteen minutes. Repeat if necessary. Call a doctor if severe.

Oncoming diabetic coma: Too much sugar, and too much fat being burned. It may come on with some other illness, such as flu. The signs are thirst, excess urine, tiredness, drowsiness, cramps, nausea; later, abdominal pains and shortness of breath. Call the doctor promptly: this is his responsibility.

WOMEN AND DIABETES

Of the 2,000,000 diabetics in the United States, 1,250,000 of them are women. Diabetic women used always to be infertile. Nowadays, with proper treatment, nearly all who want to can have babies, but they need special care during pregnancy. A low-salt diet is usually indicated to counteract a tendency to retain fluid in the tissues. An early delivery, either vaginal or caesarean, is safest for the baby—probably during the thirty-sixth or thirty-seventh week. The Mount Sinai Hospital in New York figures on more than 92 percent success in births with diabetic mothers.

Research into the causes and permanent cure of diabetes continues; but even now a diabetic who has his head screwed on right has no need to die before his time, nor must he live a life of invalidism and restriction.

FOODS HARMFUL TO DIABETICS—HIGH CARBOHYDRATE VALUE

Sugar, glucose, sweets, chocolates.
Honey, jam, marmalade, syrup, molasses.
Cakes, biscuits, pastries, puddings, pies, tarts.
Bread, toast, potatoes.
Milk puddings, Jell-O, canned fruits.
Thick soups, gravies, sausages.
Sodas and carbonated drinks; malted-milk drinks.
Beers; liqueurs; cider; all alcoholic drinks except whiskey, brandy, and dry wines.

FREE FOODS—NEGLIGIBLE CARBOHYDRATE VALUE

Tea, no sugar or milk.
Coffee, no sugar or milk.
Clear soup.
Bouillon, consommé.
Lemon juice.
Unsweetened pickles; vinegar; horseradish.
Mushrooms.
Saccharin.
Vegetables: Brussels sprouts, cabbage, carrots, cauliflower, celery, cucumbers, green beans, leeks, lettuce, onions, scallions, peas, rutabagas, spinach, tomatoes, turnips, watercress.
Fruits: Cranberries, grapefruit, gooseberries, lemons, melons, loganberries, red currants, rhubarb.

FOODS SUPPLYING
TEN GRAMS OF CARBOHYDRATE

Bread, white or brown, ⅔ ounce; toast, ½ ounce; Ry-Krisp, crackers, ½ ounce; unsweetened pastry, ⅔ ounce; oatmeal, 4 ounces; breakfast cereals, 2 ounces; corn flour, spaghetti, rice, etc., dry, ½ ounce, cooked in water, 1½ ounces; spaghetti in tomato sauce, 3 ounces; cocoa, 1 ounce; Ovaltine, ½ ounce; cream soup, 4 ounces; ice cream, 2 ounces; Jell-O, 2 ounces; fresh milk, 7 ounces; ale, 1 pint; Guinness, ½ pint; 2 lumps of sugar; potatoes, boiled, two ounces, baked or French fried, 1 ounce, fried, ⅔ ounce; baked beans, lima beans, pea beans, sweet corn, canned peas, 2 ounces; fresh or frozen peas, 4 ounces; beets, parsnips, 3 ounces; apples, 4 ounces; bananas, 3 ounces; cherries, 3 ounces; damson plums, 4 ounces; grapes, 2 ounces; oranges, without skin, 4 ounces; orange juice, 4 ounces; peaches, 4 ounces; pears, 5 ounces; raspberries, strawberries, 6 ounces; dried fruits: apricots, ⅔ ounce; prunes, 1 ounce; dates, currants, raisins, ½ ounce.

9

Your Digestive System and Liver

Your digestive system is more like a mistress than a servant. It responds to your every mood, is upset when you are upset, and calm when you are contented. It accepts what you give it and makes the best of whatever treatment it receives—and gives you pleasure every day.

Your liver, which works in association with your digestive system, is the main processing plant and general chemical works of your body, and apart from its innumerable routine roles, it operates a twenty-four-hour-a-day rescue service, clearing your blood of poisons or rendering them harmless. This applies to medicines, such as sleeping tablets, taken to act specifically for a certain time, as well as other drugs, like alcohol, certainly not taken for the benefit of your health.

Even so, accommodating and cooperative as your alimentary tract may be, it can come back at you—lethally—if you insult it sufficiently often and severely. You can die young from stomach disease, colon disease, or liver disease. Each arises in a different way, and each needs separate consideration.

YOUR STOMACH

You don't actually need a stomach. It's an anachronism, a relic from the days when to get enough nourishment you might have to snatch what food you could and cram it into your mouth before someone else got it. Carnivores, like dogs and cats, who always bolt their food, have proportionately capacious stomachs: that of an Alsatian dog holds five pints, compared with a man's modest two and a half.

The stomach is basically a storage container, so that you can fill up with food and then run—or fight. It is now also a digester and mixer. Both its massaging movements and the digestive juices it pours onto the food make the latter more suitable for the further processes of digestion and absorption in the intestines than the casually chewed chunks you send down. A unique power of the stomach is the production of quite strong hydrochloric acid (0.17N), useful for sterilizing the food when it arrives, and also for softening tough meat fibers, etc., to ready them for digestion. What is so remarkable is that the lining of the stomach can remain unaffected by the acid. Yet, as we shall see, the slightest breach will allow this acid to attack the tissues; ulcers occur only if there is acid present.

The stomach also produces pepsin, which substance initiates the first part of the process of splitting protein foods into simpler compounds. Food remains in the stomach for two to four hours, depending on type and consistency. Fatty foods, for instance, slow down the movements of the stomach and so delay the passage of its contents. The section of intestine immediately beyond the stomach, into which it gradually empties, is called the duodenum. It is only in the stomach and the duodenum that peptic ulcers may occur.

PEPTIC ULCER

An ulcer is a raw place on the lining of the stomach or duodenum usually between a half inch and one inch across; usually there is only one of them. The majority— 60 percent, and the proportion is increasing—are in the duodenum and are called duodenal ulcers, while those in the stomach, called gastric ulcers, are most often found quite near its exit into the duodenum. Ulcers frequently first start causing trouble between the ages of thirty and forty for men and ten years later for women, and once they've arrived they are likely to last, getting gradually worse over the next five to ten years. Peptic ulcers are painfully disabling, but their danger to life lies in their complications, which are hemorrhage or perforation.

About one fifth of ulcer victims suffer one or the other of these disasters, usually after they have had the ulcer for some years, and so should have been able to see the red light. Both hemorrhage and perforation are caused by the stomach acid acting on the unprotected raw tissue, by making it bleed severely or by eating a hole right through into the abdominal cavity.

There are about seven new victims of peptic ulcer per thousand people in Britain, and slightly more in the United States, every year, which makes this a comparatively common disease—and one that carries a double danger of dying young.

PREDISPOSING CIRCUMSTANCES

Men—or women past the reproductive phase—are most prone to ulcers—especially the duodenal type. The ratio for male to female is 10:1 for duodenal ulcers, and 3:1 for gastric ulcers. It seems to be a matter of those protective female hormones again, since ulcers rarely develop during pregnancy—the chances are seventy thousand to one against—when a woman is more hormonal than ever. And if a woman has an ulcer *before* she becomes pregnant, it soon heals when she is expectant.

People with blood group O are particularly susceptible to duodenal ulcers—40 percent more likely than the average to have one—and 20 percent likelier than others to develop a gastric ulcer. Apart from the blood group, heredity does have an effect on the likelihood of ulcers, and the tendency can run in a family. Acute ulcers, which sometimes persist and become chronic, may appear after a surgical operation; a shocking injury, especially a burn; or after a psychological shock—which implies that acute stress has something to do with it. Fierce emotion may well make ulcers likelier.

However, the case of the overworked executive and his "businessman's ulcer" is a popular myth. Those in responsible positions in the professional, managerial, and executive groups have only 45 percent of the average incidence of ulcers among employed males in general. Deadline tension is more likely to get you in the heart than the stomach, although bus drivers in London do get more than their share of ulcers. On the other hand, no one is immune, and statistical probability won't help if you happen to be among the still considerable number of executives with an ulcer.

Seasons have an influence, and you are least likely to get ulcer symptoms in the summer—perhaps because your meals are lighter and you take it easier. But from autumn through winter is the worst time of the year.

Various medicines can damage the stomach lining and make it bleed, paving the way to ulceration. *Aspirin* is the one in most common use, either alone or in a combined analgesic tablet with a name that may put you off the scent. (The small print listing contents—acetylsalicylic acid, salicylate, or the like—will alert you.) The worst thing is to toss down a tablet whole, because it will stick against the stomach lining. Soluble aspirin in water or calcium aspirin is the least harmful, but some stomachs, like some people, are more sensitive than others.

Phenylbutazone, given for arthritic pain, attacks the

lining of the stomach and is used experimentally *to induce* ulcers in dogs.

Corticosteroids, helpful in many conditions, can cause dyspepsia (32 percent), ulcers (7 percent), and perforated ulcers (5 percent) if they are taken in high dosage for a long time.

Antibiotics can cause vomiting but do not seem likely to lead to ulcers.

Smoking does not cause peptic ulcers—the ulcer rate went down while the smoking rate went up. But there is incontrovertible evidence that it delays the healing of an ulcer once it has developed. The situation is rather the same with alcohol, coffee, tea, irregular meals, poor teeth, infection, and worry. These don't produce an ulcer, but they may lead to relapse and deter recovery.

There does not seem to be an "ulcer type"—another myth to lay to rest. Any individual can get an ulcer, and the anxious, furrowed face and thin, dyspeptic look of the ulcer victim are the result rather than the cause of having so many miserable meals and suffering so much pain.

Apart from getting pregnant—which certainly is out for men—there is no special way to protect yourself from ulcers. If your stomach is naturally a toughie there is no need to pamper it. But if it shows signs of feeling the strain of life, then you would be wise to try, prophylactically, the course we recommend as a postulcer regimen.

SYMPTOMS TO AROUSE SYMPATHY FOR YOUR STOMACH AND/OR DUODENUM

Discomfort or pain above the navel, sometimes also in the lower chest or the back, which tends to come on directly after a meal might mean that a gastric ulcer is in the offing; if the pain comes on two to three hours after a meal it might indicate duodenal trouble. It is characteristic of duodenal ulcer that it wakes you in the small hours with pain.

Milk, an antacid, or vomiting relieves the pain, by diluting, neutralizing, or getting rid of the acid. It is the effect of the stomach acid on the raw part that produces the pain.

Your mouth may fill with fluid for no apparent reason.

You may get heartburn—a burning sensation behind the breastbone—often at night.

Your doctor, to whom any of these symptoms should have sent you, will probably confirm the ulcer diagnosis by arranging an X ray and an occult blood test on your bowel movements (all ulcers bleed slightly). If necessary, endoscopy—passing an illuminated tube into your stomach —may be done.

IF YOU HAVE AN ULCER, OR ARE IN DANGER OF ONE

Your doctor will take over. The main weapons he will use on your body's behalf will be:

Rest: For your body in general, and you may also have to face actual bed rest—for your mind, for that controls your bodily peace, and specifically, for your stomach.

Diet: There is a variety. For the early stages your doctor will have his own well-tried favorite.

Drugs: Antacids; sedatives; antispasmodics; and perhaps the licorice derivative carbonoxalone, which heals gastric ulcers but not duodenal ulcers: it can put awry your water balance.

No smoking order—of course.

POSTULCER REGIME

To keep you out of trouble, you should continue with it for two years at least, and go back to it for a month or two every year thereafter to give your stomach some kind of a vacation. Use it at the first hint of dyspeptic trouble.

There are two factors which need control:

The acid factor: Important but often exaggerated. The time schedule and the constituents of the diet suggested will diminish acid production in the stomach and also maintain a barrier (a creamlike fatty coating) in the stomach.

The motor factor: Probably of even greater import than the acid factor. Excessive and irregular churning and squeezing of muscles in the stomach wall may push the blood away from the surface (like your white knuckles when you clench your fist) and so make the mucous lining more susceptible to the effects of the acid. Or the over-vigorous movements may force the food against the stomach wall and damage it by both the impact and the rubbing. Lastly, if an ulcer is present, or if the tissues are on the point of breaking down to form one, they need rest from movement if they are to mend, like a cut or wound anywhere. The diet suggested in the following pages is one that calms rather than stimulates the movements of the stomach.

GENERAL RULES

1. Never go for more than two hours or so without food. Arrange to have a milk drink and a cracker in midmorning, midafternoon, and at bedtime.

2. Have three main meals a day, with the snacks mentioned in between; or have four meals, plus a midmorning and bedtime snack.

3. Take your meals at regular times each day.

4. Take your time over them: be like Mr. Gladstone and chew each mouthful thoroughly, if not thirty-two times as he did.

5. Don't dash around just before or just after meals: even a few minutes' rest ante- and postfood is beneficial.

6. Get enough sleep to wake rested.

7. Don't be persuaded to have a large meal, a fried

meal, or any food or drink that you know disagrees with you.

8. Avoid foods that are very hot, very cold, chemically stimulating, or mechanically irritating—there is a list of these later on in the chapter.

9. Give up smoking, but if you can't, confine it to the period after a meal, when your stomach is well lined.

10. Never drink alcohol before meals, when the stomach is empty.

11. Drink sparingly with your meals, as this will ensure proper mastication; but have plenty of water between meals.

12. See your dentist regularly.

STARTER'S DIET

For when you are just coming off your doctor's prescribed diet or at the first hint of dyspeptic trouble.[1]

ON WAKING
Glass of milk from allowance[2] or weak tea with milk and sugar if you like.
Cracker or ½ slice of crisp toast, buttered when cold.

BREAKFAST
Strained oatmeal with milk from allowance, or small helping of cornflakes (avoid cereals containing bran, fruit, or nuts) with fruit purée, juice, or milk from allowance.
1 egg or small piece of white fish.
Crisp toast, buttered when cold, or buttered bread at least 24 hours old.
Jelly, marmalade, strained honey.
Weak tea or coffee (decaffeinated) with milk from allowance and sugar as desired.

---

[1] From *Human Nutrition and Dietetics* by Davidson and Passmore.
[2] Allowance for day: 1 quart of milk.

MIDMORNING

Glass of milk from allowance, or milk drink.
Cracker.

LUNCH

Strained cream soup, if desired.
Small helping of fish, lean, tender meat, or chicken.
Strained vegetables.
Potatoes, mashed or creamed, or crisp toast.
Milk pudding with strained fruit, or mousse, or gelatin
made with fresh fruit juice, or soufflé, with cream.

MIDAFTERNOON

Crisp toast, buttered when cold, or day-old bread made
into sandwiches with sieved hard-boiled egg, scrambled egg, finely minced chicken or ham, or cream
cheese.
Jelly, strained honey.
Plain sponge cake, Madeira cake, or crackers.
Weak tea with milk from allowance and sugar as desired.

SUPPER

Egg, or cream or grated cheese, or meat, or chicken, or
fish, as at midday. Strained vegetables if desired.
Small helping of milk pudding with fruit purée, or fruit
purée and cookies, or lunchtime sweets. Bread and
butter may be substituted for the sweets.
Weak tea or coffee with milk from allowance and sugar
as desired.

BEDTIME

Milk drink and crackers.

When your stomach has settled, take a more liberal
view. Still stick to the rules but check what you eat and
drink by the O.K. and "watchit" lists below.

O.K.

Dairy products: Milk, cream, yogurt, butter, cream cheese, eggs—except fried.

White fish: Steamed, baked, boiled, grilled.

Meat: Sweetbreads, brains, tripe, chicken, rabbit, lean ham, tender beef, mutton, lamb.

Crisp toast, buttered when cold; rusks; white bread, not fresh.

Plain biscuits and crackers, plain cake, sponge cake.

Honey, jellies.

Cereals, refined and well cooked, such as corn flour, semolina, ground rice, oatmeal.

Junkets, gelatin, custards, blancmanges, soufflés, mousse.

Potatoes, boiled, baked, and mashed; green and yellow vegetables finely strained and puréed with butter.

Fruits, stewed and finely strained, served as purées, and fruit juices strained, sweetened, and diluted for drinking, or used in gelatine.

Weak, milky tea or coffee. Choose a decaffeinated brand.

WATCHIT

Alcohol, strong tea and coffee, gravies and soups made from meat extracts.

Raw vegetables, cucumbers, celery, onions, radishes, watercress, tomatoes, mushrooms.

Raw unripe fruit; dried fruit (currants, raisins, prunes, etc.); nuts; seeds, skins, and peels of all fruits whether cooked in puddings, jam, or cakes.

Pickles, condiments. Spices are probably harmless.

Tough, twice-cooked, or highly seasoned meats, including sausages, bacon, pork.

Fried fish, fatty fish such as herring, kipper, mackerel, salmon, sardines.

Rich or heavy puddings.

Fried foods in general.

Fresh bread, scones or cakes; hot, buttered, soft toast; whole-meal bread or biscuits; rye or wheat Melba toast; coarse cereals; cakes containing dried fruit or peels.

BOREDOM IS THE BUGBEAR
OF THE ULCER DIET

When you are planning or choosing a meal out consider these possibilities:

Eggs: Your best standby. You can have them scrambled, boiled, poached, baked, shirred, coddled, or in an omelet; and graduate to omelets with various sweet and savory fillings; and then to Oeufs Niçoise, and Oeufs à la Reine.

Soups: These must be home-prepared or made by a first-class chef from *basic ingredients,* not flavored extracts. A grinder or blender is essential. Suitable varieties are potato, carrot, and bean soups; cream of pea, mushroom, watercress, and asparagus soups.

Fish: May be poached; creamed; served in egg sauce; baked; casseroled; boiled; made into a soufflé; graduate to fish pie, grilled fish, and Sole Bonne Femme.

Meat: Try lightly grilled liver; creamed sweetbreads; grilled chicken breasts; chicken casserole; shepherd's pie; broiled chopped steak; grilled filet mignon.

Pasta, rice and cereal: Cook fresh for each meal, tender but not soggy. Useful in soups or with meat. Top it with melted butter; margarine; salad oil; warm milk or cream; cream cheese; cottage cheese; vegetable purée. Later: olive oil, tomato purée (homemade), and herb butters.

Vegetables: Best pressure-cooked, and the fluid kept for soup or a cold drink. They can be mashed, puréed, served in white sauce or soufflé, or mixed with potatoes, pasta or cereal. Potatoes baked in their jackets are good; scoop out the soft center, mash with cream or butter, and pile in again—add vegetable juice or purée sometimes.

Sweets: Milk puddings; gelatin sweets; Jell-O made with ¾ milk; baked and boiled custards; caramel cream; mousse with chocolate or fruit purée; soufflés; baked bananas; baked apples; meringues; Bavarian creams; angel food cake; pound cake.

BLENDER MEALS

Your best investment, once you realize you have a tendency to ulcer, is a food blender. Any food that has been through the blender will be smooth enough to be acceptable to the most delicate stomach.

THREE BLENDER MEALS
(BLEND EACH FOR ½ TO 1 MINUTE; SIP)

Start with a cup of milk, a cup of cream, and an egg for each recipe. Add:

1. 4 ounces orange juice, 1 teaspoon instant decaffeinated coffee.
2. Half a ripe banana, 2 tablespoons instant cooked cereal; 1 tablespoonful of honey. Have the milk warm to start.
3. 3 ounces tomato juice; 2 tablespoons wheat germ; 1 tablespoonful melted butter.

The blender is also invaluable for making sandwich spreads, e.g., cream cheese and chicken breast; diced roast beef and egg; fish, carrot, and egg; hard-boiled egg and cottage cheese. All should be moistened with salad oil.

It may be a bore to keep an ulcer tendency under control and to treat your stomach with consideration, but this is a sure way of avoiding dangerous and deadly complications. However, in the more liberal diets you must avoid overnourishment and the resultant overweight, as this is as dangerous to you as to anyone else. And when you are quite well, cut down on the animal fats—cream, butter, cream cheese—and use plenty of cooked fruit in your diet: even an ulcer candidate can get a coronary. Exercise (not just before or, more particularly, just after a meal) is important to keep your heart and circulation in good condition.

TROUBLE BELOW: COLON AND RECTUM

Your stomach receives, stores, and partly digests your food. Your small intestine—twenty-two feet of it—completes digestion and absorbs what is valuable to your body; the food is also taken to the liver for further processing. What remains in your bowel is useless or unabsorbable, and includes a great deal of bacterial debris (you defecate even if starving) which is washed down with water into the large intestine or colon. This is wider than the small intestine but only about four feet long.

The colon starts in the lower right-hand corner of your abdomen, and at this point it has a fingerlike, blind-alley off-shoot, the appendix. The rest of it is festooned loosely around the edge of the abdomen, mainly, until at the lower left-hand part of it, it becomes the rectum, or back passage, ending in the anus. The colon conserves fluid for you by absorbing about half a liter of water from the waste material in it, so that this waste can be stored fairly compactly for evacuation once a day—on the average—unlike urination, which is relatively frequent. The colon produces mucus to lubricate the evacuations. The rectal section of the colon is sensitive, and when it is full you are aware of the fact; it will set off a reflex wave of muscle contraction throughout the colon, which should empty its total contents all at once.

This is how the system is *meant* to work: neatly, efficiently, trouble-free. But like other good systems, it can go wrong, and particularly if it isn't used in the way intended. There are various disorders of the colon in modern civilized man, all interconnected. The most dangerous of these is *cancer of the colon, including the rectum:* this kills more men than any other cancer, with the exception of lung cancer. What makes one wonder where we are going wrong is the fact that there is more cancer of the colon in the United Kingdom and the United States than anywhere else in the world, although the advanced countries of Europe come close.

Of 49,000 cancer deaths in Britain in 1969, 15,000 were due to this kind of cancer. The figures were significantly *lower* a few years ago: 14,500 in 1965, 13,500 in 1935. Treatment, by a complicated surgical bypass, often leaves the patient with the embarrassing handicap of being unable to use his natural anus, and, moreover, is by no means always effective. The five-year survival rate for this cancer, after operation, is 21.4 percent, and only two thirds of this figure for ten-year survival.

Early detection helps with any form of cancer, but with this one more than most, since there is an 80 percent cure rate for those cases caught before the growth has spread outside the bowel wall.

In the United States in particular, screening programs at cancer detection centers provide for just those examinations that will discover this kind of cancer or its possible precursors: polyps of the colon. *Sigmoidoscopy* is the passing of an illuminated tube into the rectum as far as the S-bend of the colon: no anesthetic is required. A *barium enema,* in which the colon is filled with a radio-opaque material and then filmed, will reveal abnormalities farther up the colon—but these are less common. Both of these procedures can be performed in a screening. You *must* have them done at the slightest hint of trouble.

SIGNS TO SEND YOU AT ONCE
FOR EXAMINATION OF YOUR COLON

1. Bleeding from the rectum. This may signify piles, or piles and some other trouble higher up.
2. A change of any sort in your accustomed bowel habits that continues for more than a week.
3. Slime, with loose or frequent movements.

These three symptoms could mean trouble low in the colon or rectum. The next three could mean trouble in the higher reaches:

1. Constipation. This is very common anyway.
2. Fullness and flatulence.
3. Colicky pain, often on the right side.

With either trio you may feel run down, and find yourself anemic.

It may save your life to find a precancer through screening, or by a prompt reaction to symptoms. If a precancerous condition—say polyps—is discovered, and an operation suggested, don't hesitate: think of it as a lucky opportunity for safeguarding yourself. The discovery is equivalent to the situation in which a woman who has a precancerous condition of her cervix has it brought to light by the Pap smear. Both situations give people a chance to stop cancer before it has begun.

AVOIDING COLON DISEASE

A stitch in time is clearly worthwhile. It is obviously better if the stitch doesn't ever become necessary, because that means that the damage has been avoided. And it looks as though this is now possible. Appendicitis, diverticulitis, polyps of the colon, cancer of the colon, and two rare ones, ulcerative colitis and regional ileitis, are all disorders affecting the same colonic area and apparently associated in some way with the Western life-style.

Denis Burkitt, M.D., F.R.C.S. Ed., already world-famous for his work on Burkitt's lymphoma, believes that these diseases, in common with obesity, diabetes, atheroma, and dental caries, are caused by the faulty diet of modern, highly industrialized man. The association between dietary factors and these "diseases of civilization" is as clearly defined, he says, as that between smoking and lung cancer.

Let's take a look at the evidence: it is vitally important to those who prefer survival.

Appendicitis has been common in the West ever since King Edward VII made it fashionable at the beginning of this century, when food processing was first getting under way. Now it is the commonest emergency operation among Americans, white and Negro equally. Yet appendicitis is almost unknown among blacks in rural Africa: its incidence has increased tenfold during the last twenty years in many *cities* in Africa, however. It is also becoming more and more common in Americanized Japan, while the Japanese who settle in the United States are as liable to it as native Americans.

Diverticular disease of the colon, which consists of little pouches off the colon, is so common in our civilization that 20 percent of all the apparently normal, healthy people in Britain can be seen to have diverticula on X-ray examination. Europeans and Americans from the United States living in the tropics are forty times as likely to have diverticular disease as the native population. In our society, middle-aged women who have had children are particularly liable to this common condition.

Ulcerative colitis and regional ileitis (Crohn's disease) are rare colon disorders which affect young adults. Both of these disorders carry a definite predisposition to cancer of the colon, and both seem to crop up almost entirely among the industrialized peoples.

Polyps of the colon: These growths of the colon are not in themselves harmful, but are in time likely to develop malignancy. Apart from a hereditary type—familial polyposis—polyps are found in 20 percent of people over the age of thirty in Britain and America, shown by autopsies performed after accidents, etc. Yet polyps simply don't occur in the colons of people in economically underdeveloped communities.

Cancer of the colon occurs about equally among whites and Negroes in the United States. It doesn't affect Negroes in rural Africa at all, and so far only a few cases have appeared in African cities. It takes twenty years to induce a cancer of the colon, so one can see the natural time lag from the effects of "civilization" in action in Africa. Cancer of the colon is also rare in Japan, but the incidence rises dramatically a generation after emigration to America.

It seems plain that there is something in the Western way of life that tends to produce diseases of the colon.

It appears to have something to do with our diet: low-roughage, high-sugar, high refined-flour content. No people living on the opposite diet of high roughage, low sugar, etc., is affected. Our diet produces a small stool bulk, since there is less of unabsorbable plant fiber in it. This in turn means that there has been a slower transit time, and a longer storage of stools in the body until there is enough to stimulate evacuation; also, the stools are more viscous. The result of this is increased pressure inside the bowel to move the relatively constipated material along, and it is this pressure that is thought to be the cause of appendicitis, diverticula, and polyps. Any cancer-inducing substance in the bowel will remain in contact with its walls longer than if the diet were more stimulating. It has also been suggested that the bacteria which are present in the intestines of people on our kind of Western diet may manufacture carcinogenic substances.

Other "diseases of civilization" which we have mentioned—diabetes, obesity, etc.—are forty times commoner in urban Africans than in those in rural areas. It seems that a concentrated-sugar, refined-carbohydrate intake may throw a strain on insulin production and lead to diabetes through exhaustion of the pancreas. Again, the small volume of our sweet and concentrated foods leads us to crave more than is sufficient to nourish us if we are to feel satisfied; this of course is the root cause of much obesity.

Dr. Burkitt's conclusion is that in the West we are all living on a deficient diet: deficient in the unabsorbable roughage that is necessary for a healthy colon. The diet is also excessive in sugar and refined carbohydrate.

So it looks as though the call is "back to nature," and that to avoid most modern colonic troubles, from constipation to cancer, we should aim at a diet like this one:

ON WAKING
Glass of hot water with lemon juice.

BREAKFAST
Coarse oatmeal porridge, bran cereal, or Birchermuesli, with dried or fresh stewed fruit, or sliced banana, or grated apple. No sugar added. Milk, if desired, but not cream.

Egg, bacon, fish, or liver with tomatoes.

Whole-meal bread, oat cake, or bran muffin with coarse-cut marmalade. Fresh fruit. Tea or coffee as desired, with milk, no sugar.

MIDMORNING
Apple, pear, other fruits in season. Any drink.

LUNCH
Vegetable soup, including plenty of chopped fresh vegetables, dried peas, beans, lentils, and barley.

Meat or fish, with generous helping of vegetables, or, frequently, salad. Potatoes cooked unpeeled and eaten peels and all: not too much.

Fresh or stewed or grated raw fruit with cookies, or pudding made with dried fruit and/or nuts.

Oatcakes with cheese. Coffee with milk if desired.

MIDAFTERNOON
Sandwiches made with whole-meal or rye bread, filled

with dates and walnuts; cheese and apple; lettuce, tomato, cucumber, cress, either plain or with egg; or whole-meal bread or rye or wheat Melba toast with preserves or comb honey.
Gingerbread, fruit or nut cake, coconut cookies, etc.
Tea with milk.

DINNER
As lunch; one of these two meals may be lighter than the other.

BEDTIME
Glass of hot water, flavored if desired.

Take liberal quantities of raw salads and coarse green vegetables, as well as other vegetables; fresh or cooked fruit; nuts. Don't peel anything unless it is absolutely necessary. Don't strain the pieces out if you make lemonade.

And, as with all diets, cut down if you find yourself getting overweight. Since well-trained abdominal muscles help keep the colonic muscles inside toned up, involve yourself in some regular exercise that uses your abdomen: almost all sports do. Unless you add *butter and other fats* to this diet it is conveniently low in atheroma-producing fatty foods.

CIRRHOSIS OF THE LIVER

In Britain, men in administrative and professional jobs have twice the national average incidence of deaths from cirrhosis, possibly because their higher incomes allow for a higher consumption of alcohol. In the United States the situation is worse: cirrhosis is mounting in the charts as a cause of death, and it is not confined to any groups, since presumably more people there can afford to become regular, substantial ingesters of alcohol.

Cirrhosis is a slowly advancing strangulation of the working cells of the liver by scarlike tissue. This process, unless it is halted, leads inevitably to death, for there is almost no chemical transaction in the body that does not depend upon the liver in some way.

PREDISPOSING CONDITIONS

In the United States especially, chronic overuse of alcohol is the commonest factor in the development of cirrhosis. Alcohol can poison the liver cells directly. Ninety to 95 percent of the alcohol you drink means work for the liver, which must oxidize it into carbon dioxide and water. Even a single large dose of alcohol can damage the liver of a healthy man, at least temporarily, and occasionally jaundice or frank inflammation of the liver may come on after a drinking bout. So it is not surprising that long-continued, excessive use of alcohol can lead to long-term liver damage. Both wine and spirits can have this effect.

Alcoholism can also indirectly affect the liver, because a drinker often consumes a diet that is deficient in particular food materials which are essential for the health of the liver: these materials include the B group of vitamins and some protein constituents. The harm wrought by dietary deficiency on the liver can be seen in the pathetic pictures of protein-starved children of Africa with the disease called kwashiorkor, with its terribly swollen livers.

However, you don't *have* to be an alcoholic or be visibly starving to develop cirrhosis. It can come on for no discernible reason, and is perhaps more likely if you have ever had an attack of virus hepatitis.

SIGNS THAT YOUR LIVER MAY BE UNDER THE WEATHER

1. Vague digestive complaints, actually caused by congestion: flatulence, nausea, lack of appetite, vomiting—and all of these are typically worse in the morning.

2. You may, later on, have pain under your ribs on the right side, and feel distended, which may be due either to gas in your intestines or to collecting fluid.

3. You are likely to be pale and actually anemic.

4. You have rough skin, and a smooth tongue.

5. You have "spider marks"—made up of blood vessels; warm palms of the hands; a tendency to bleed easily.

6. You may have a bluish tinge to your face, or it may be slightly browner than it used to be.

AVOIDING CIRRHOSIS

The obvious thing to be avoided is alcohol. Alcohol is a pleasant social lubricant, a relaxer of tensions, and a promoter—as a rule—of good fellowship. It acts by depressing the higher nerve centers, and so its first effect is to reduce the sense of worry, and so to bring about a feeling of well-being. But even in small doses it impairs the judgment and inhibits the skills necessary for fine movements—without the drinker's being aware of any change.

It is understandable that during or after a period of stress a person may slip into the habit of dependence on this valuable social drug. The trouble is that it is addictive, like any other drug that makes you feel good, and it has the added danger of easy availability. The time to stop being an alcoholic is before you have begun, while you can still go without a drink for a whole day without missing it. If you find this difficult, it is time to take stock. If you find it impossible, or find that you need a drink before breakfast to get you started off on the right foot, it is time to get professional help. See your doctor.

If you are unlucky enough to catch virus hepatitis, as thousands do, make sure you convalesce completely, so that your liver is back to 100 percent before you take another drink.

When there is a yellow warning from the above symptoms, go for tests and treatment from your doctor. The liver cells will regenerate and further fibrosis may be prevented, liver reserves may be built up, and fluid retention, if any, stopped—particularly if you start treatment promptly and stick to it.

There may be nothing specific you need to do. In that case, you can pamper your liver by a high-protein, moderate-fat diet, like this one.[1]

DRINKS
Anything but alcohol.

ON WAKING
Tea with milk, sugar if desired—or fruit juice with sugar.

BREAKFAST
Oatmeal or cereal or stewed fruit, with milk; or fruit juice.
Lean bacon, grilled and drained of fat; or egg, not fried; or piece of fish; tomato.
Bread or toast, butter, marmalade, or honey.
Tea or coffee with milk.

MIDMORNING
Coffee with milk. Cracker.

LUNCH
Large helping of lean meat, poultry, liver, kidneys, tripe, sweetbread, lean ham, white or smoked fish.
Vegetables and potatoes, not fried.
Light pudding made with egg; fresh, stewed, or canned fruit.
2 plain crackers with cheese.

MIDAFTERNOON
Sandwiches filled with egg, cheese, minced meat, or ham.
Small piece of plain cake, or plain cookie.
Tea with milk.

---

[1] *Op. cit.*

SUPPER

Average helping of meats suggested for lunch; or egg with lean bacon (not fried); or 2 eggs scrambled; or cheese. Vegetables, if desired. Milk pudding and fruit, or bread and butter and jam.

Coffee with milk.

BEDTIME

Milk drink. Plain cracker.

Take each day: 1 pint of milk, 3 ounces of butter, *no more*. Don't eat fried foods, pastry, pies, heavy puddings.

10

Women in Particular

A woman has some things a man has not: breasts and a womb, for instance. These may be her strength in some ways, but they are definitely weak spots in terms of survival. In almost every other area man is more vulnerable than his mate, but a negligible number of men die from breast cancers, and none at all, of course, from cancer of the womb, or from the side effects of the pill. These are the hazards of femininity.

BREAST CANCER

In Britain, eighteen thousand women a year develop breast cancer and ten thousand die from it—an average of thirty-one a day. The figures are proportionately greater in the United States, and they have been rising slightly over the last ten years. Among women in the West this is the commonest cancer, accounting for 20 percent of all cancer deaths. It affects the comparatively young, the forty to forty-nine age group.

The highest breast cancer rate in the world is in Denmark, while it is very low in Japan and Chile, where cancer of the womb is more of a plague.

ASSOCIATED FACTORS— PERHAPS PREDISPOSING

The highest risk of breast cancer is among the following: nuns; unmarried virtuous spinsters; women who have had no babies, or mothers who have never attempted to breast-feed; women continuously on the pill for two or more years; women who have had breast trouble in the past, such as mastitis, nodularity, etc.; women over thirty-two; and women in the highest social class.

WHAT HAPPENS

A cancer of the breast, like any other cancer, is a gang of cells that have got out of control and continue to multiply madly, not only when there is no purpose, but when their presence is actually doing harm by crowding out the normal working-cell population and invading their territory. The original, tight-packed mass of malignant cells in a lump is the *primary tumor*. Secondary tumors, or metastases, can crop out if some of the cancer cells become detached from the main site. They may travel to some distant part of the body, say the liver, in the bloodstream, and settle there; or they may reach the lymph glands near at hand via the lymphatic channels. It is the secondary tumors that constitute the risk to life.

It seems that the background situation for the development of breast cancer parallels that underlying the male cancer of the prostate gland, and that there is often some abnormality in the balance of the sex hormones. At any rate, the breast is normally greatly influenced by hormones from the hypothalamus, the adrenal glands, and above all the ovaries, and it is significant that breast cancer will regress—temporarily—in 40 percent of those cases in which the ovaries are removed.

Basically, a breast cancer is a lump in the breast, but not all lumps in the area are cancers: they may be cysts, part of a generalized cystic hyperplasia, or a small area of fibroadenosis.

PREVENTION

Marriage and four breast-fed children constitute one preventive measure.

The second is regular self-examination of the breasts, from age thirty, say four times a year, always just after a period, perhaps on the seventh day after the first day of flow. Be systematic: lie on your back, a flat pillow under your upper chest and shoulders, and nude above the waist. Rest your left hand above your head and with your right hand examine the whole of your left breast, part by part, starting in the upper outer area. It is important to use the flat of your hand to feel with. Change over and use your left hand to examine your right breast.

This examination is well worth doing. Dr. Charles Gros of Strasbourg says, "It takes years to become a good palpator. But women know their own breasts, and may notice a lump, pain, or excretion that a doctor might miss. I myself would have missed many lumps shown to me by patients."

Of course, if you think you have detected a lump, or even some irregularity of texture in your breast, report it to your doctor *promptly*. Similarly, let him know if you have a pain in the breasts not confined to the time just before a period; or a discharge from the nipple; skin trouble around the nipple; alteration in the appearance of the breast; or swelling of the breast.

The third sensible precaution against cancer that every woman should take is a triennial or annual—if advised—

screening, at a center equipped for the task. The whole procedure takes no more than an hour and a half, and goes something like this:

Completion of a short questionnaire covering general health, past and present; any previous breast trouble; pre-period discomfort; babies and breast feeding; periods and any troubles with them; any other troubles in this area; and whether you are or have been on the pill. You are also asked about your family and any serious disease among near relatives, and any particular problems or worries you may have.

Clinical examination: A medical carried out by a gynecologist, of which the important parts are the examination of your breasts and abdomen externally and of your womb, ovaries, etc., internally. A cervical smear is taken—that is, a spatula is rubbed across the neck of the womb to pick up a few cells from the surface for microscopic study. A sample of the fluid in the vagina may also be taken. Blood pressure is checked, and blood taken for a test.

Laboratory investigations: The cells from the cervix are assessed for abnormality, particularly for changes that could be precancerous. Samples from the cervix and vagina are also cultured; that is, added to materials suitable for bacterial or fungal growth, and then studied to see what infective organisms, if any, can be found. A blood test discovers whether or not you are anemic, and is an indirect check on the seriousness of any undue blood loss.

Thermography: This is a method of making a picture of the warmth of the various areas of your breasts, using an infrared detector. The actual temperature scanning takes only five minutes, but before that you have to sit around for ten minutes in an air-conditioned room, bare from the waist up. The skin temperature may also be studied with thermistor probes and infrared photography. The aim is to discover any areas hotter than the rest, which might indicate some infection, or possibly unusual activity in the cells which might tend toward cancerous change.

Mammography or senography, its sophisticated big sister, is a special kind of X ray of the breasts. It is useful when the thermograph is difficult to make out and the doctor's examination has been hampered, for instance, by the size of the breasts. Not all cases require mammography.

VALUE OF SCREENING

Although the detection of precancerous conditions is the main purpose of this type of well-woman screening, they are by no means the only unsuspected troubles which may come to light, which is to the benefit of the patient. Anemia, for example, may be sapping a woman's vitality without her knowledge: this would be discovered by the routine blood test.

A cervical smear can forewarn of the possibility of cancer up to *twenty years* in advance: the suspect tissue can be removed at this stage without even preventing the woman from having more babies if she so wishes. In the few cases in which a cancer has already begun to develop it is likely to be still in the bud stage, and easily, safely, completely removable. Other, less dangerous, abnormalities may be found in this area: erosions (cracks), polyps, and infections of the cervix; vaginal infections; fibroids of the womb, and cysts of the ovaries.

Breast examination may reveal a coarse-grained, even knobby texture to the tissue. This is found in nearly half of all women taking the pill, but it almost always clears up in a few months if the pill is discontinued, and it may not necessarily come back after a return to the drug. Cancer is more common in a nodular breast, however, which should make any high-risk woman, perhaps one whose mother had a breast cancer, think favorably of some other type of contraceptive. Others would do well to "surface" from the pill for two or three months every year, as a precaution.

At present, three out of five breast cancers are not diagnosed until they have already spread beyond the breast and are difficult to cure, but in 70 percent of cases of breast cancer picked up through screening, not even the nearby glands in the armpits are affected. For a woman, breast and cervical examinations lessen the worst dangers to her life and should be regularly done.

AT THE WORST

One of the things that makes some women hesitate before being screened for cancer is the fear that if one is found it means a certain, painful death sentence. In this day and at this stage of medical advance neither is likely to be true. Early treatment offers a good chance of cure. It may involve:

1. Removal of part, or more likely the whole of one or both breasts. Don't let this dismay you. What else are falsies for?
2. Radiation treatment, with or without operation, for some types of cancer only.
3. Hormone treatment, usually in addition to 1 or 2. There are new drugs being introduced against cancer, notably ICRF-159, which appears to prevent the secondary growths which do most of the damage, and immunity treatments similar to those used in Austria by Dr. Issels also hold promise. Even if cure should prove impossible, modern treatments can prolong your life and improve its quality.

CANCER OF THE WOMB

Fifty years ago cancer of the womb was commoner than cancer of the breast, but now it is only half as common. Nevertheless, thousands of women die young each year from this kind of cancer. There are two kinds: cancer of the cervix, or neck of the womb, and cancer of the body of the womb. The former is twice as common as the latter.

FACTORS ASSOCIATED WITH CANCER OF THE CERVIX (PERHAPS PREDISPOSING?)

Early start to sex life; a full sex life with changing of partners; several children; marriage alone doubles the risk; a confinement multiplies it by ten; usually occurs past thirty but especially around fifty (but it will have started years earlier); Negroes are particularly susceptible; it is commoner in large cities, seaports especially, than in small towns or in the country; wives of over-the-road truck drivers, men in the services, and others who are away from home for days on end are susceptible; widows and, more especially, divorced women are susceptible; it is commoner among the less skilled than among professional workers or the wives of the latter.

It is obvious that cancer of the cervix is in some way connected with coitus, yet fewer than 2 percent of married women get the disease. It is known that married women produce agglutinins against the sperms of their own spouses—a type of immunity reaction. Changing of partners may set this mechanism awry. Jewish women are practically free of cancer of the cervix: perhaps this is a matter of race, perhaps it is because their husbands are circumcised. There is some evidence that smegma, the material from under the foreskin, may have some relationship to this form of cancer. It is less likely when the man uses a condom regularly or the woman a diaphragm, and if the man is careful of his cleanliness or is circumcised.

AVOIDANCE OF CANCER OF THE CERVIX

Since living like a nun isn't likely to be appealing, and besides, it increases the risk of breast cancer, statistically speaking, a compromise is to avoid promiscuity or use a barrier-type contraceptive for any irregular sexuality. Most important of all: *have a regular cervical smear.*

This can be conveniently fitted in with a breast check, in a well-woman screening program previously described, or it may be done alone. Microscopic examination of the cervical cells can reveal precancerous abnormalities, which are a warning of danger ahead if nothing is done. It can also reveal what is known as a *cancer in situ,* one that has not begun to invade the surrounding tissue and, like precancerous conditions, causes no symptoms, and cannot be detected by the doctor. It can be removed with a certainty of cure.

Even a developed cancer of the cervix, discovered early, as by screening, carries a 70 percent chance of a five-year cure—one assumed to be complete—while at the later stage the chances of cure drop to 7 percent.

Symptoms that should lead you to seek advice include any abnormal discharge from the vagina after intercourse, on passing water or moving the bowels, or at other times; and unusual bleeding, from spotting to flooding. Of course, there are other, less harmful, reasons for such symptoms, such as polyps or endometriosis, but a gynecological check at the first sign may prevent you from dying young.

FACTORS ASSOCIATED WITH CANCER OF THE BODY OF THE WOMB

This type of cancer is less common, cannot be picked up by a smear test years in advance, and arises in women about ten years older than those with cervical cancers. It goes with overweight; stocky build; one or more children —though 30 percent of those afflicted have had none; fibroids; diabetes; delayed menopause, which may be five years past the average age of forty-eight; and heavy and irregular bleeding at the menopause.

Symptoms that should lead you to have a checkup include bleeding, as we have mentioned, and even more, if such bleeding comes after the menopause; discharge, often like dirty water; difficulties with passing water, you do so too frequently, have an urgent need to, and lack full control; and pain low in the abdomen. As with cancer of the cervix, these symptoms may be due to a less serious cause, but checking up is common sense. Luckily the wall of the womb is singularly resistant to the penetration of any growth inside it, so treatment is likely to be completely effective if taken early.

Treatment for both types of cancers of the womb may combine operation and radiation, and the sooner the safer. Like being caught for speeding by a police car on your tail, there's no excuse for letting a cancer in this area catch up with you and do you dirt. It is a matter of going regularly for smears from, say thirty-five on, and reacting promptly to any untoward symptoms.

The importance of special screening for women cannot be overstressed. In a program carried out in 1970 in the London borough of Ealing, 23 percent of the apparently fit participants were shown to be in need of some kind of treatment to benefit their health and comfort. Among four thousand women seen, twenty-six cases of unsuspected cancer were picked up. Women are fortunate that their weak spots are so clearly seen in screening.

THE PILL

The contraceptive pill is revolutionary: the first method of birth control, apart from sterilization, that is virtually 100 percent effective, and that moreover involves no preparation at the time of intercourse. No wonder that its popularity was so great that twenty million women were taking it in 1969. In Australia and New Zealand one third of married women under forty-five are on the pill, in the United States over a quarter of them, and in Britain about one sixth. The most successful and commonly used pill—there are several different variations on the formulation—

is a combination of the two chief female sex hormones, estrogen and progesterone.

The pill usually prevents the monthly release of an ovum, or egg cell, from the ovaries, but it also makes pregnancy impossible in other ways. It changes the chemical constitution and the consistency of the mucus at the mouth of the womb, so that sperm are no longer welcomed, and it alters the way in which the lining of the womb is built up, so that it is no longer prepared to receive a fertilized ovum.

The pill has been around for about sixteen years, and in that time, with so many using it, a few hazards have come to light. Only a small minority of women are affected, but it is not always possible to tell in advance who these will be. The occasional dangers of the pill include:

Jaundice: Occasionally a woman may have this indication of liver disturbance—yellow skin, eyes, etc.—shortly after starting the pill. It is known that steroids, which the pill hormones are, can disrupt liver function: it is the estrogen component that is probably responsible. Usually the jaundice rapidly disappears if the pill is stopped, so the danger is more apparent than real, unless the liver is already damaged.

Thrombosis and embolism: Thrombosis, the spontaneous clotting of blood, usually in the veins of the legs, is eight times more likely to happen to women on the pill than to others. The danger of this clotting is that a small fragment of the clot may become detached and carried in the bloodstream until it ends up blocking a small artery elsewhere in the body. A clot lodging in the lung, pulmonary thromboembolism, may cause sudden death in a young, healthy woman (see Chapter V). Or the clot may form in the brain, with equally disastrous results—cerebral thrombosis is six times as likely when a woman is on the pill. It is still, of course, rare. Also, a coronary thrombosis may occur more easily.

Again, it seems that the estrogen part is the compound responsible. Estrogens given to men, for instance in the treatment of prostate disease, have been found to have similar effects on the blood-clotting factors in the blood and have a tendency to induce spontaneous thrombosis. A satisfactory progesterone-only pill would sidestep this particular hazard, but those tried have had other disadvantages and dangers.

It is not merely a matter of the constituents of the pill itself, however: the woman's own make-up has an influence. For instance, those of blood group O, the commonest in the United States and the United Kingdom, run only one third the risk of pill-associated thromboembolism. The risk of thrombosis is greater, however, over thirty-five. One to two women in every 100,000 die from thrombosis brought on by the pill every year, among the under-thirty-fives. Four women in every 100,000 die among the over-thirty-fives. *But* about twenty-four women in every 100,000 of those pregnant die of thrombosis every year —and maybe some of them would not have become pregnant if they had been using the pill. However, the pill may be taken year in and year out, while pregnancy lasts for nine months and usually occurs only a few times in a life.

High blood pressure: This is only occasionally associated with the pill. In a study of fifteen hundred American women on the pill none had a higher blood pressure than before. However, when it does occur it seems bound up with the production of renin from the kidneys (see Chapter VII).

Cancer: There has been a continuous and close scrutiny for any connection between cancer and the pill, but this is somewhat hampered by the fact that the induction period (between cause and development) in most cancers is about twenty years. A connection with cancer of the breast is hinted, however, by the finding at screening clinics that women on the pill have a coarsening of the texture of the breast tissues such as is sometimes seen in breasts that develop cancers. The doctors who run screening clinics include in their "high-risk" groups for breast cancer those who have been continuously on the pill. This is about the same rating given women who have shown an abnormal thermogram.

A similar, unproven correlation has been suggested between the pill and cancer of the cervix.

Diabetes: Alterations in glucose tolerance, possibly predisposing to diabetes, are quite commonly found among women on the pill.

UNWANTED EFFECTS OR SIDE EFFECTS FROM THE PILL WHICH POSE NO DANGER TO LIFE (MORE THAN 50 PERCENT OF WOMEN HAVE NONE)

Reduction in the supply of breast milk.

Reduction in fertility: some women find that their periods do not return on giving up the pill, others that they do not conceive within the usual three months after breaking off.

Increase in weight (may right itself after a few months).

Depression, irritability.

Headaches.

Nausea—usually only in the first two months.

Breakthrough bleeding; a change of brand usually helps.

Loss of libido—but, on the other hand, some gain.

Heavy feeling in breasts, premenstrual tension.

Worsening of varicose veins.

All in all the pill may not be the best contraceptive for you if you have, or have had: thrombosis; liver disorder, unless in childhood only; high blood pressure or kidney disease; depressive illness, severe enough for medication or hospitalization; or breast trouble.

And if you *must* take the pill—it has much to offer in peace of mind and convenience—come off it, as I have already urged, for two or three months every year, to allow your system a respite from the all-pervading effects of the hormones it contains.

BEYOND THE CRUNCH

VIRGINIA WATERHOUSE: BREAST CANCER

Ginny was forty when it happened, on the young side of the average for such things. Her husband was in the export trade, and she wrote novels—rather sentimental stuff but easy to read and steadily salable. They had one child, Clandon, who was away at school.

Ginny was quite careful about her health and on her fortieth birthday went to the local clinic, which was offering free cervical smears for a two-week period. Oddly enough it was when she was drying herself after a shower that evening that she noticed it: a small firm lump, like an almond, deep in the outer quadrant of her right breast. For three weeks she did nothing, hoping that it might magically vanish, but it did not. She saw her doctor.

After that, things moved. The doctor referred her to a surgeon, who performed a biopsy—an operation to sample and identify the structure of the lump; it was a cancer. The surgeon explained to Ginny that this would necessitate a *radical mastectomy:* complete removal of the affected breast and some of the underlying muscle. There was no choice between this and waiting for it to grow and spread. So Ginny agreed.

She was in the hospital for two weeks. It was when she was nearly due to come out that the depression swept through her. She felt that her life as a woman was over, and like "a bird with broken wings." Her husband cared. He hired a physiotherapist to help and guide her through the physical difficulties of an arm inclined to swell, weaker than it had been, and with the fingers awkward to manipulate. He insisted that she have the best prosthesis available—the sort you can swim with, and so realistic that even a child cannot detect the difference in a cuddle. He took her on a holiday somewhere they'd neither of them been before. And he made their first act of intercourse a bridge to emotional healing. From an intimate and satisfying sex relationship Ginny drew much of the courage she needed to face a future inevitably somewhat shadowed with uncertainty.

Ginny has written her first best seller, some four years after her operation. No one outside the family remembers, no one would guess at her encounter with cancer, but to Ginny it has added a depth of understanding, and given her a new context of values.

11

Mind!

Like every other living creature, you and I are primarily concerned with our personal survival and—probably—our reproductive performance. Because we cannot achieve either in isolation we have to maintain a working relationship with our environment and the others who share it. As we are all in the same situation, with similar aims, this must involve some competition and some cooperation.

Stress is a state of preparedness for such cooperation and competition. It is obviously essential to our existence, but those who survive will be the ones who learn how to handle it, without incurring damage. Disease is an unsuccessful attempt by the body or mind to adapt to its circumstances. It took two hundred million years for mammals to evolve from fish, but it has taken man only ten thousand years to come from the Stone Age to the space age. In the last hundred years we have increased our speed of travel a hundred times, the power of our weapons a million times, and our speed of communication ten million times. Our cities—crowded multitudes of strangers living together—impose undreamed-of stresses, and neither our minds nor our bodies are built to cope with them.

The body may respond with a recognized disease reaction. In the advanced and affluent countries, where these new stresses are greatest, characteristic diseases are coronary disease, high blood pressure, diabetes, gallstones, ulcerative colitis, cancer of the lung, and traffic accidents. Hypertension certainly seems to be associated with social stresses: it is a major killer in industrialized Japan, yet almost unknown in the Pacific Islands nearby; it is common among the blacks in the northern cities of the United States, yet rare in people of the same stock in Africa. Peptic ulcers and tuberculosis are unusually common among the widowed and divorced, a reflection, perhaps, of the effects of loneliness. Asthma, migraine, hyperthyroidism, and appendicitis are more frequent among those who live under stress.

As well as the bodily diseases brought on by stress, it has obvious and sometimes devastating effects on the mind, and it is not surprising that 45 percent of hospital beds in the West are occupied by the mentally sick. Psychological disturbances can also kill you.

Suicide, car crash, accident: all are dramatic ways of dying young, and all are caused—at least in part—by a state of mind. Anxiety can inch your blood pressure up and release extra cholesterol into your bloodstream, with attendant atherosclerotic dangers. Or the highly competitive business world, the deadlines, and the frequent need to be in two places, geographically distant, at the same time, may call for a quality of sustained performance that may psychologically tax a man—or woman—beyond the limit of his or her capability in the end; particularly since home and marriage, in this divorce-ridden age, and children, in this era of militant youth, are likely to be an added source of tensions, rather than the haven of security they once were.

Suicide is the ultimate in succumbing to stress, and, like sex, it is presently popular. Even more popular than complete self-destruction are "suicide bids," which are a means of communication. It is a cry for help, sympathy, rescue from an unbearable situation, or love, if a person takes an overdose of drugs sufficient for an urgent rush to the hospital but not sufficient to run a great risk of death.

Sometimes such maneuvers misfire. The dose is judged incorrectly or help arrives on the scene too late, so this can be a dangerous game that sometimes ends up the wrong way. It usually does not succeed in its aim anyway, as it has become so commonplace as to be regarded as a troublesome bore rather than a high tragedy by other people. The woman who crammed a handful of sleeping tablets into her mouth, staggered to her ex-boyfriend's door and said, "I've come to die in your arms," didn't die—or get the man back.

Apart from those suicides which come off in spite of the victim's intentions, there are yearly thousands of others which are absolutely intended, mostly among men. Despair over some personal disaster, the feeling that every exit is blocked, or a hopelessness that sweeps over one in unreasoning waves may put a person into the kind of mood that some quite minor event could trigger into suicide. Reasonable precautions against doing something irrevocable in time of stress are these: avoid keeping drugs or firearms available; keep in the company of other people when you are low, or at least stay in telephone contact with them, and seek your doctor's advice if you find yourself harboring thoughts of suicide. Antidepressants work miraculously for some kinds of miseries, and there is always some sort of help for other kinds.

Although you may put aside guns and throw away sleeping pills, you are certain to keep in constant use today's most common lethal weapon: your car.

CAR CRASHES

A car crash can be one form of suicide. A Harvard Medical School Research Project on fatal highway collisions concluded, after examining 125 fatal "accidents," that no fewer than nine were deliberate suicides, and four were unpremeditated acts. There's no one so likely to indulge in this form of suicide as the man who is furious with his wife as he goes around a blind corner—this is a form of Russian roulette.

There are other attitudes of mind that are forerunners of car crashes: outlets for pent-up aggression; expressions of virility, especially among males with a Latin streak; hunger for thrills in a workaday existence; depression, so that one doesn't care; elation, so that judgment is too optimistic, perhaps due to alcohol or pep pills; drowsiness or fatigue from narcotics or from driving too long; or disruptions of the body's time system (e.g., as when one who normally retires at eleven is on the road at three in the morning).

The plot thickens when you consider that a man in a car is like a centaur, with different powers and a different psychology from his pedestrian self. When you are in the driver's seat you are armored and partly mechanized, and also cut off from a number of your normal bodily and mental inhibitions and safety devices. My meek and elderly aunt, who almost apologizes for her existence, is a ruthless, determined being when she is coupled to her car. The man who is basically not confident and unsure of his attractions and powers is likely to change personality in a car and become a brash, overconfident exhibitionist.

The car itself may contribute too much to the combined man/vehicle system, so that the man may not be fully in control. This situation was recognized by Judge Glenn Sharp of Oklahoma, who let a motorist free but had his car impounded after he had had an accident.

You—and all other drivers—encounter a new situation with new dangers as soon as you sit in your car. In your walking life your complex nervous system, with its feedback and automatic correction devices, protects you. However overweight, you are unlikely, for instance, to misjudge the size of a gap that you can get through. If you are on uneven ground, or begin to stumble, you automatically adjust your balance and save yourself. I don't suppose many people have actually fallen over since they were three.

But as that bio-robot, the man in a car, you don't automatically come to a halt if something goes wrong. And you don't even get a stomach ache if some mechanical fault is developing. Your powers of self-regulation in movement, which took millions of years to evolve, don't operate on wheels. If you put your foot down on the ground in walking, messages flow back to your brain and down to your foot continuously; but when your foot presses an accelerator or a brake pedal you have no such information service or any certainty of the consequences of your actions.

In a factory the machinery has built-in safety devices so that if a worker makes a mistake the machine either stops, corrects the fault automatically, or operates a signal to attract the attention of someone who will put it right before any harm results. An automobile has no such saving mechanism. It depends on the individual attached to brake, clutch, and accelerator. According to Aldous Huxley, the relationship between a man and his car is much what it may be between a man and his dog: it must subserve him absolutely, making him feel like a small god. A car inflates a man's self-esteem, adds to his social dimension, makes a nobody into somebody, empowers him to do things outside his normal range—all this in competition with others.

A car, like a gleaming coat of mail, is a symbol of potency, prowess, and invulnerability (however false this all may be)—and, for a woman, of elegance. A car, like a child, is an extension of yourself, but is a good deal more obedient. It is not just sitting in your car but the way in which you maneuver it that gives driving all this symbolic significance; yet you have an odd anonymity in a car. Just as when you are on vacation abroad, with no friends watching you, you may release your inhibitions and do as you wish in a manner that is out of the question in your office or home, so can you act in a car. You can let your temper come to a boil and let out a little of it; you can be selfish—or daring.

The saying that a man "drives as he lives" is manifestly untrue. Driving brings out elements normally suppressed or concealed under custom's mask of courtesy and consideration. Of course, this may only apply to the "other" drivers. You may have nothing but loving-kindness within you, but it is more likely that there is undiluted aggression. Aggressivity is an instinct that wells up spontaneously. It is a biological necessity for a cornered animal, or for survival in the business world, or for winning a mate. Various inborn and trained-in inhibitory mechanisms prevent us from hitting or biting each other in irritation, but these won't check your foot on the accelerator. The deep emotions of personality don't register the damage you can do to yourself or others by so trifling a movement.

Present-day civilized man suffers from insufficient opportunity to discharge his aggressive drive. That this is directly connected with deaths by automobile is borne out by two facts. One is that women, although no more skilled than men at manipulating a car, have proportionately far fewer accidents (231 males per million are killed on the roads in Britain, compared to ninety-one females): women are less aggressive. Secondly, the Ute Indians, in whom aggression has been bred, have a higher rate of car accidents than any other group.

Consider the situation: the roads filled, and filling further, with herds of bio-robots which have the powers of machines and the aggressions of uninhibited men. The whole scene is fraught with occasions when irritation is inevitable and reprisal, or at least vigorous reaction, is only natural. But it nearly always takes two to make an accident, just as it takes two to make a quarrel or love. If one won't play it's that much safer. You can be that one.

A moral veto is no good against an instinctual drive, but a simple ploy is to satisfy your aggressive feelings outside of your car. This will not only have the effect of reducing your liability to road accidents, as you will be less likely to react to aggression *with* aggression, but it will also help sidestep the feelings of anger and frustration that contribute to coronary and blood pressure disasters.

Take every opportunity of releasing your aggressions on a physical plane through sports, and if you don't want to get involved too competitively try horseback riding, skiing, skating, swimming, gardening, sex, long-distance running, or mountaineering—though this last carries high hazards of its own. Sports are not only an outlet but an education in the responsible control of your drive.

Sublimate some of your fighting spirit in creativity: carpentry, building a pool, making music, conducting a business, writing a book.

Express your feelings vicariously with loud music, live theater, spectator sports.

Above all, cultivate the antidote: laughter. Humor is the latest human characteristic to develop—our grandfathers had precious little of it—and it is *uniquely* human. It is developing rapidly nowadays as a sign of culture, especially in the United Kingdom and the United States. It enables you to appreciate—for the primitive antics they really are—the behavior of other drivers whose instincts have deflected their judgment, and to laugh at them as well as at those who are just plain stupid. If you can occasionally laugh at yourself you have reached the highest achievement of civilized man, and have attained the complete safeguard against inner arrogance.

You may decide to invest in psychoanalysis, with a view to having your personality overhauled, with the undesirable elements taken out: an expensive but popular pastime in some circles.

This is background care, but at the moment of truth, when you are just setting off in your car, consider these points:

1. Start sooner than you have to. If you don't, have someone phone and say that you may be late. This takes the tension off.

2. Patch things up with your wife or colleague before you make a move: in the long run it'll save time and maybe your life.

3. Have your radio on to keep you entertained and in a pleasant mood in traffic jams and to shut out your problems in transit.

4. Sing.

5. Don't add to your tensions and reduce your capabilities by dictating letters, etc., en route, unless of course you have a chauffeur.

6. Get in a merry-go-round mood: when you are on the golden gallopers at a fair it is the motion, not the speed or the getting somewhere, that makes it enjoyable: enjoy the city or country you are driving through.

7. On a long trip take a break every hour and a half.

8. Shout and swear at the other fools, whenever you want.

9. Take a companion whenever possible.

10. Remember that the greater your skill and experience, the greater your need for prudence. British racing driver Mike Hawthorne died in a car crash the day after he had retired from racing, and when he was both fresh and sober.

You are more likely to react slowly or mistakenly in certain circumstances:

1. When you are tired. A five-minutes nap on the side of the road is better than eternal sleep prematurely. Have a cup of coffee to help the revival process.

2. When you have had a tranquilizer, or an antihistamine pill (for instance, for hay fever), or an antidepressant. However, if your doctor has prescribed these, knowing that you drive, you probably operate better when you have had them. Travel-sickness pills are never necessary for the driver of a car, but be cautious if you drive off a ferry after having taken sickness pills for the crossing.

3. When your blood sugar is low. Don't miss meals when you are traveling; or suck a cube of sugar. Don't put yourself to sleep with a heavy meal.

4. When there is carbon monoxide in the atmosphere, as in a polluted city or, more especially, when you smoke a cigarette while at the wheel. Carbon monoxide in the blood first impairs your concentration and increases irritability, then makes you headachy, dizzy, confused, and nauseated.

5. When you have had alcohol. Alcohol in moderate dosage does not decrease your driving skill, but it wrecks your judgment; you would not be aware of this.

6. When driving outside your normal time schedule.

This can affect you the same way that alcohol or fatigue affects you.

Illness: Accidents due to a driver's sudden illness at the wheel are rare—say one in a thousand, but more may be precipitated by a driver's being under par. The onset or convalescent stage of flu; high blood pressure; diabetes; epilepsy; coronary disease; and blackouts from any cause should make you consider having a medical check before you drive. But disease is less deadly than arrogance on the road.

The few accident-prone individuals are not responsible for the majority of fatalities. Ordinary drivers, when they are careless, preoccupied, tired, or bad-tempered, cause 90 percent of the crashes and suffer 90 percent of the deaths.

Practical factors: Regular servicing of your vehicle, with special attention to the braking, lighting, and steering systems, is an obvious precaution. Check your tire pressure and the state of the treads frequently. Get small faults corrected promptly and unusual sounds or symptoms diagnosed. Probably the greatest single life-saver is wearing a seat belt which provides all-around protection.

IT HELPS TO GROW UP

Car drivers involved in fatal or serious accidents per 100,000,000 miles driven:

Age Group	Number Involved
Up to 19	410
20–24	204
25–29	134
30–39	104
40–49	95
50–59	75
60–69	75
70 and over	147

JET SET

It is a mark of success to be frequently in demand, in person, in multiple places an air trip apart. Jet travel has added a new dimension to living, and it needs correct handling for you to get the best results from it while risking your neck—or heart—the least.

Firstly, are you fit for jet travel? If you are near fifty, fat, and smoke, you should have an electrocardiograph to make sure you never had a silent or an indigestion-pain coronary in the past; a hemoglobin check to ensure that you can stand up to reduction in oxygen pressure; and a blood pressure check.

Aircraft cabins are pressurized to the equivalent of an altitude of about five thousand feet. Any reasonably fit person should find it no strain on his heart and arteries to sit in a seat at this height, or to stroll up and down the aisle, although strenuous exercise might be a different matter. But if you are traveling to somewhere like Peru or Nairobi you will be landing higher—atmospherically speaking—than you were flying, with a greater chance of running short on oxygen.

If you are a smoker, for instance, part of your hemoglobin, the oxygen-carrying compound in your blood, is out of service in the form of carboxyhemoglobin, the carbon monoxide derivative. A smoker at sea level has to live as though he were at five thousand feet; at five thousand feet as though he were at ten thousand feet. If, for any other reason, your hemoglobin is less than 100 percent—a diet without enough emphasis on iron and vitamin C, or bleeding piles, for instance, or if your breathing apparatus, which is responsible for taking in oxygen, is impaired, you may be in a delicate situation. Your heart muscle may feel the pinch for oxygen; any chest trouble will feel worse; and your brain power will take a dip: you will be less alert, feel fatigued.

This will all be aggravated by either alcohol or loneliness.

A reasonable precaution would be to quit smoking for a few days before your trip, in order to improve your oxygen-carrying capacity. Changes of pressure may upset your digestive system and give you spasms of pain or wind. This is an unpleasant but not serious effect and calls for simple foods, no alcohol, and, if you expect it in advance, anti-peristaltic tablets from your doctor.

The physical effects on the arteries to the heart and brain of sitting cramped and still, and the attendant increased danger of a coronary or a stroke, have been discussed earlier. The other aspect of jet flying is the psychological stress of putting your life into a craft over which you have no control, and from which there is no possibility of getting off en route, and the exhausting effect on your nervous system of the continuous noise and vibration. A tranquilizer may cushion you from these effects, but not everyone needs this. You may revel in the stimulus of travel, or by now be completely bored.

Everyone, however, is subject to jet-lag fatigue. This is a genuine condition, not a phony excuse for bad decisions made by executives abroad. We saw, in Chapter IV, that your body runs something like a silent symphony orchestra with its various functions all keeping to their own rhythms, yet all in harmony. Your temperature, for instance, ordinarily peaks at 10 P.M. and takes a dip at 2 A.M.; you produce less urine at night, regardless of what and when you drink; the electrical activity of your brain and circulation and your multiple chemical processes—all are subject to individual rhythmic variation every twenty-four hours.

A trip into another time zone may bring the strain of being suddenly plunged into a new culture and a new climate, as well as a new time. If your bodily rhythms are out of phase, this alone is enough to decrease your mental acuity by 5 percent. A businessman flying from London to New York, leaving at 10 A.M., will arrive 1 P.M. local time. But for him it is already 6 P.M., and it has been a tiring day. His organism cries out for dinner, relaxation, and bed. He is crazy if he has lunch and an afternoon business conference instead. At least one prominent industrialist was accused of being drunk at a board meeting when he had not had a drop, but was simply jet-fatigued.

We have all seen politicians showing unaccustomed hesitation and inarticulateness in press conferences televised immediately following intercontinental flights. Such situations are enough to give anyone a stroke—literally.

The traveling businessman can expect to feel better and to give a significantly better performance if:

1. He travels with a congenial companion, and works with at least one colleague with whom he is on friendly terms when he arrives.

2. He takes an adequate rest after arrival. One major oil company, not noted for extravagance, instructs its long-distance travelers to do no work during the twenty-four hours after arrival.

3. He travels by day whenever possible.

4. He eats and drinks sparingly on the way.

5. He gets to bed as soon as possible on arrival, irrespective of local time or entertainments. He may need a mild hypnotic, perhaps one alcoholic drink, to help him get to sleep.

STROKE

Stroke causes 12 percent of all the deaths in Britain and North America, counting third among the killers, after heart disease and cancer. Suddenly, a part of the brain is put out of working order, due to a disaster in an artery supplying it. The functions of the brain that can be disturbed in this way include the control of movement, sensation, speech, understanding, and emotional control. There are three types of stroke:

Cerebral thrombosis: The cousin of coronary thrombosis, and, like this, caused by the spontaneous clotting of blood in an artery damaged by atherosclerosis (deposits of fatty material in the arterial wall). Both are very much on the increase, but the difference is that cerebral thrombosis tends to crop up later, at fifty-five plus, rather than at forty plus. This is the commonest form of stroke.

Cerebral hemorrhage: The cracking and leaking of a narrow, stiffened brain artery. It tends to come on earlier than thrombosis, at fifty to seventy, and has a particular association with high blood pressure. At the end of the Second World War it was far commoner than thrombosis, but now the positions are reversed.

Cerebral embolism: The sudden blocking off of an artery by a fragment detached from a clot elsewhere, usually the heart. This is the least common type, and comes, as a rule, even earlier: in the forties.

A serious stroke of any of these types can kill you outright, cripple you, or give you timely warning to take care for the future by special health measures. Transient cerebral attacks and minor strokes, producing only temporary symptoms, are particularly valuable as signposts and spurs to action.

CAUSES OF STROKE

It is partly a matter of constitution. If your parents had strokes this is a possibility you should consider in relation to yourself, so that you can take evasive action. High blood pressure, your own or in your family, is a factor to heed as a warning. However, there is no inevitability about following in your father's footsteps, just a somewhat greater chance unless you take care. If you are constitutionally fat you are that much more susceptible to stroke, but not as much as if you have recently acquired a middle-age spread. If you are a man you are more likely to get a stroke: the ratio is three men to two women, up to the age of seventy.

PERSONAL PREDISPOSING FACTORS

Smoking: Stroke is three times as common in smokers as in nonsmokers, and ten times as common if one also has high blood pressure and a high level of cholesterol in the blood. People who have had repeated small strokes often stop having them when they stop smoking, and they come again if the smoking starts again. The more heavily you smoke the worse off you are.

Smoking also tends to give one a taste for salty and spicy foods, and this may have some indirect effect on liability to stroke.

Overeating, particularly of fats and sugar, in relation to your physical activity, and especially if you used to be slim, is dangerous. The habit of drinking milk instead of water with meals is deplorable. Milk *is* a meal. Besides, too much animal fat—milk, eggs, cheese, butter, cream, meat fat, lard—can lead to a raised blood cholesterol count, which is a risk factor in itself.

Inactivity: Stroke is less common among postal delivery-men than among clerks in the sorting office; among bus conductors going up and down the stairs of London's double-decker buses than among drivers; among those whose work involves their muscles than among desk work-ers. And those who have a long sleep at night increase their risk of stroke.

Even after one stroke, a second stroke is less likely among those who make every effort to remain active.

Stress or long-term tensions and an anxious reaction to the demands of life are also factors in stroke. Neither physical nor mental work produces the stresses that can lead to stroke, but worry, frustration, and suppressed anger may. The shock and frustration of retirement or demotion is a not uncommon forerunner. A personal disaster may have an immediate effect. Henry II of England, who never smiled again after his son Prince William went down in the White Ship, probably had had a stroke and couldn't smile. Winston Churchill had his first recognizable stroke when he tasted the bitterness of losing the first post-war election in 1945. The coming to light of a long-hidden, shameful secret has more than once brought on a stroke.

Dr. Alan Barham Carter, a British expert on stroke, considers the stresses of modern jet travel a contributing factor in the disease; he has found unduly high blood pressures among fit young men who had been jet test pilots. The two major precipitating factors in stroke are a stressful situation and a shortage of fluid. The latter could stem from sweating excessively, but the classic occasion occurs when a businessman has flown five thousand miles to attend a conference which he anticipates will be sticky, and has had a couple of stiff drinks to steady himself first. Concentrated alcohol withdraws fluid from the blood.

Other disorders which may predispose to stroke, apart from atherosclerosis and high blood pressure, which are its essential basis, include diabetes, thyroid deficiency, gout, kidney disease, and rheumatic heart disease. There is effective simple treatment available for the first two, and at least worthwhile treatment for the others.

HOW NOT TO HAVE A STROKE

1. Cultivate a tolerant, patient, relaxed, adult attitude in the face of annoyance or antagonism, on the golf course as much as at work. It is a sign of immaturity to get steamed up at every setback or irritation. Ride it out.

2. Accept as inevitable some limitations to your business activities, and have *genuine* vacations (not on the firm) and occasional afternoons off to be with your family. On the principle of breaks for soldiers on the march, you will travel farther this way.

3. Don't smoke, or if you must, cut down.

4. Use some polyunsaturates in your diet—margarine on your bread or corn oil in cooking.

5. Use your muscles. This uses up calories in the form of fats and sugars. It calms you emotionally and gives you a snug sense of physical well-being. It directly benefits your circulation.

6. Don't miss out on sex: the exercise equivalent of a brisk five-mile walk, a tranquilizer, and a stimulus to the glands that keep you youthful—all these are to be found in the sex act.

7. Watch out for the yellow warning signs, below, and remedy them if they appear.

Health farms are helpful as far as they go, but two or three weeks of expensively healthy living, once or twice a year, doesn't make up for living the major part of your life in an unhealthy way. It takes *four months* to reeducate your tastes and habits, if they need it. However, you can do nothing but good to yourself at one of these special social establishments.

YELLOW WARNING

"Coming events cast their shadow before," sometimes. Signs that your cerebral arteries are narrowing significantly include transient attacks, lasting a few minutes or occasionally as long as an hour, in which a limb is weak or the fingers are suddenly clumsy. It may be a momentary feeling of confusion, or the wrong word slipping out unexpectedly; you may have pins and needles on one side, although you haven't been lying on it, attacks of dizziness, or disturbance of your vision. Any of these may indicate some fleeting interference to the circulation to the brain and should send you to your doctor to find out what is going on. It may be nothing.

Increasing thirst and increasing output of water combined with a loss of weight could be due to diabetes; check.

Slowing up, gaining weight, and feeling the cold unduly could mean thyroid deficiency; check.

Acute pain and swelling in a joint, especially the big toe, may mean gout; check.

LITTLE STROKES

These show that the arterial difficulties in the brain have arrived at a ticklish stage. Little strokes comprise an interference with brain function, lasting hours, or perhaps a day or two, with the same type of symptoms as with transient cerebral attacks. It is commonly on waking up that the victim finds to his surprise that his hand has "gone to sleep" or that one leg is too weak to hold him when he tries to get up. Sometimes there are several little strokes before a serious one.

MAJOR STROKE

Today's most common thrombotic type usually occurs in your sleep: you open your eyes feeling dazed—you may have had a period of unconsciousness—and find yourself paralyzed perhaps down one side, and unable to speak properly. Cerebral hemorrhage produces a sudden severe headache, vomiting, and then coma, while embolism comes on most suddenly of all, with immediate loss of power and often of speech.

AT THE CRUNCH

The first part of managing a stroke case depends on doctors, nursing, and the family. But as soon as you realize that you have had a stroke your task is to make a continuous, maximal effort to use the powers you have and to learn new ways to manage, despite those powers that are lost, temporarily or permanently. This should be done even though you would prefer to let others do it all for you. If a stroke doesn't kill you before you have even had time to realize it, you have a good chance of making a marvelous recovery if you use your determination from the outset. It may take a year. Physiotherapists and a speech therapist may help you.

After your stroke you will obviously be in danger of another unless you do something about it. What you *must* do: *stop smoking; keep slim; keep active;* mind your blood cholesterol by avoiding eggs, butter, cream, and meat fat; don't lie in bed for more than a seven-and-a-half-hour stretch, nor sit still for long periods; and avoid anxiety and anger. Your doctor will probably help by giving you anti-coagulants to discourage your blood from clotting, and antihypertensives to keep your blood pressure in check, if necessary.

LOUIS PASTEUR, 46: SEVERE STROKE

Over a matter of about thirty-six hours a paralysis gradually affected Pasteur's left side and became permanent, and he was unable to speak. His speech returned after two days, but he thought he was dying. He made a slow recovery and lived for another twenty-eight years. It was during this time that he formulated his most famous and important theories on immunity and vaccination. His stroke was certainly not the end of his useful existence. He died ultimately of heart and kidney failure.

WALT WHITMAN, 39: MILD STROKE
FOLLOWED BY OTHERS MORE SEVERE

After his at first mild and subsequently severe strokes, Walt Whitman continued making notable contributions to American literature until his death—from tuberculosis of the lungs—at age seventy-two. A propensity to stroke neither diminished him intellectually nor caused him to die particularly young.

WINSTON S. CHURCHILL, 74: SEVERE STROKE

Churchill's first transient cerebral attack was in 1945 when he lost the election, and he had a major stroke in 1949. He made a good recovery, although already in his mid-seventies, and won the next election, in 1951. He retired in 1955 and died ten years later.

12

Survival—For What?

These are dangerous and exciting times. The tide of change is at the flood. We live in an era of impermanence, when the old institutions—marriage and family, possessions, and position in the world—are becoming increasingly temporary. Fashions and life-styles are adopted and discarded, knowledge is acquired and outdated, ideas are used up sooner and faster than ever before.

It is as though we were living in the middle of a fast-breaking news story, the sort that a journalist knows will change its meaning and its shape as rapidly as he gets the words on paper.

Survival depends on keeping your head on your shoulders and your feet on the ground. You need your bodily health, your mental balance, and a sense of direction. We have been studying the art of survival mainly in terms of practical measures against the physical hazards of disease, faulty diet, unhealthy habits of living, and today's particular stresses. This must be the essential basis, for without bodily survival there is nothing. But in these swirling seventies man's age-old problems of relating to his environment are less material and more social. We in the West are no longer battling for the tangible necessities of food and shelter. We are grappling with the new ills of affluence.

Malnutrition has been replaced by epidemic obesity and diabetes.

Hard and laborious work has been replaced by sedentary occupations and their particular perils of sudden death from coronary disease.

Factory smoke and dusty working conditions have given way to personal pollution by the cigarette.

Unequal educational opportunity has been transformed into universal educational mediocrity and a lessened chance of fulfilling one's highest potential.

Infectious and poverty-linked illnesses have given way to a wave of emotional disorders.

Lack of mobility has changed to restlessness, monoxide poisoning, and the loneliness of being lost in a crowd.

Our great cities are not integrated communities but multitudes of strangers living together.

Yet, in the confusion and uncertainty of this stirring age, life can be sweet and satisfying and purposeful. You need not only bodily health but social health also.

"No man is an island entire of itself," said John Donne, the seventeenth-century poet. It was never more true than it is in this crowded century. We have to live together, work together, learn together, and help and support each other and our society. Our happiness depends upon obtaining our social needs, which are:

To relate to other human beings.

To belong to a group.

To have friends at work and away from work.

To be accepted by our acquaintances, neighbors, and people in general.

To find a personal niche in society in which to develop our own special potentials.

These are the real values in life, without which it goes sour. I would not wish for anyone I cared about merely a life of prosperity and security: these things are bound to betray us. I would hope instead that he would attain achievement after difficulties; have struggle and adventure; and possess the emotional strength to enjoy every challenge, to ride out every storm. For emotional recharging every person needs a home: a place where he or she can find and cultivate strength for striving, courage for the acceptance of the inevitable, however unpleasant, and inner peace. A home should be a resting place where vitality is restored, and today, as always, the prize of greatest virtue in it is the durable love and affection of the family, which makes survival so infinitely worth the effort.

INDEX

Index

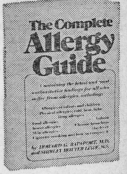

How to stay healthy all the time.

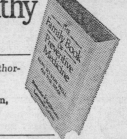

> *"I can recommend this book for authoritative answers to questions that continually come up about health and how to live."*—Harry J. Johnson, M.D., Chairman, Medical Board Director, Life Extension Institute.

Wouldn't it be wonderful if your whole family could stay healthy all the time?

It may now be possible, thanks to PREVENTIVE MEDICINE. This is the modern approach to health care. Its goal is to prevent illness before it even has a chance to strike!

A new book called **THE FAMILY BOOK OF PREVENTIVE MEDICINE** shows how you can take advantage of this preventive approach, and make it an everyday reality for yourself and your family. More than 700 pages long—and written in clear, simple language.

TELLS YOU ALL ABOUT THE LATEST MEDICAL ADVANCES

For example, the new knowledge of risk factors in disease is a vital tool of preventive medicine. With it, your doctor might pinpoint you as, say, a high heart attack risk *long before your heart actually gives you any trouble*. He could then prescribe certain changes in your diet and habits—perhaps very minor ones—that could remove the danger entirely. This would be preventive medicine at its ideal best! But even if a disease has already taken root, new diagnostic techniques can reveal its presence earlier than ever before. And, as a rule, the sooner a disease is discovered, the more easily it is cured.

SEND NO MONEY—10 DAYS' FREE EXAMINATION

Mail the coupon below, and **THE FAMILY BOOK OF PREVENTIVE MEDICINE** will be sent to you for free examination. Then, if you are not convinced that it can help you protect the health of your entire family, return it within 10 days and owe nothing. Otherwise, we will bill you for $12.95 plus mailing costs. At all bookstores, or write to Simon and Schuster, Dept. S-53, 630 Fifth Ave., New York, N.Y. 10020.